GW00502401

MULTIPLE SCLEROSIS

MULTIPLE SCLEROSIS

Exploring Sickness and Health

Elizabeth Forsythe   MRCS, LRCP, DPH

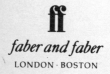

faber and faber

LONDON · BOSTON

First published in 1988
by Faber and Faber Limited
3 Queen Square London WCIN 3AU

Photoset by Parker Typesetting Service Leicester
Printed in Great Britain by
Richard Clay Ltd Bungay Suffolk
All rights reserved

British Library Cataloguing in Publication Data

Forsythe, Elizabeth
Multiple sclerosis: exploring sickness and health.
1. Multiple sclerosis
1. Title
616.8'34   RC377
ISBN 0-571-13979-5

Contents

Preface   vii

Part One

Chapter 1   My Story   3

Part Two

Chapter 2   MS – the Disease   27

Chapter 3   Investigations and Diagnosis   37

Chapter 4   Treatment and Management of MS   43

Chapter 5   Diet   49

Chapter 6   Physiotherapy and Physical Fitness   66

Chapter 7   MS Fatigue and its Management   71

Chapter 8   Acceptance of MS   76

Chapter 9   MS and the Family   85

Chapter 10   Sexuality and MS   90

Chapter 11   MS and Work   94

Chapter 12   Management of Special Problems   98

Chapter 13   MS and its Mental Effects   104

Chapter 14   Doctors and MS   107

Part Three

Chapter 15   Exploring Sickness and Health   113

Appendix   Sources of Help   139

Acknowledgements   145

Index   146

Preface

I wrote *Living with Multiple Sclerosis* ten years ago in 1977 and it was a fairly orthodox book medically speaking. At that time I wrote as a medical practitioner, journalist and patient. When, in 1985, I was asked by my publishers to prepare a second edition I intended to update the original book. However, in December 1986 I had a relapse of my multiple sclerosis and during the next two years my way back to health has been so unorthodox that I have no longer been able to do a simple revision of my original book. I have been fortunate because Faber and Faber have allowed me to write a different book and in the last part to write of some of my own new and medically unorthodox ideas.

The book is divided into three parts. The first part is an account of my own illness; the second is divided into short chapters on subjects including the disease, its diagnosis and management, with advice on diet, rest, exercise, physiotherapy, work, sexuality, holidays and problems with the family; the third part is about my own experiences of healing in the past two years and my personal ideas about MS and sickness and health.

Part One

Chapter 1 My Story

For people who have multiple sclerosis and for their families and relatives my story may be familiar. The diagnosis of MS was first made in 1976 but looking back before this I had had many health problems which could probably be attributed to MS; and like others with MS my life and health over many years had been affected by this strange disease which takes so many forms.

I was born, brought up and educated in the south of England and spent my teenage years there during the Second World War. I trained to be a doctor at a London medical school and with the benefit of hindsight I now believe that the first episode of MS occurred in 1950 during my final medical examinations. Until that day in May I had had abundant energy and managed to pass all my examinations, even collecting a prize, with a minimum of hard study. I spent a lot of time in the wards and out-patient clinics because I always enjoyed 'real' work with patients rather than book work. Life in those days seemed good with plenty of friends and a great variety of interests and activities.

And then that May day, within sight of the end of the final examinations, my left leg gave way and I was not able to get to my last clinical examination. I can now look back and think that it could not really have been so incapacitating and that with more courage and determination I could have managed somehow. I am quite certain that I was not malingering but of course the cause could have been other than MS. I had a prolonged period of rest and my leg recovered but I did not regain my earlier energy, my ability to do well in examinations and survive the hurly-burly of life in hospital medicine.

Until that time it had been taken for granted that I should stay on in the hospital world and train to be a specialist, probably in children's medicine. Although I was given a good 'house' job in general medicine at my teaching hospital I was never able to cope properly. In those days

3

we were on call every night unless we managed to do an exchange with another young resident doctor. I was just not able to cope with that sort of pressure and became so exhausted that I had to have time off work. The confidence of senior doctors in my ability waned and perhaps even more importantly so did mine. I struggled through the first six months and at the end did not get the children's house job at my teaching hospital. The reference from the senior consultant physician for whom I had been working said all the things about my distinguished student years and that my work was good and I 'took unending care of my patients'. But it ended 'perhaps her only fault is that she is over-conscientious and tends to wear herself out in the performance of her duties'. That was undeniably the truth and a damning remark; and it stopped me getting any of the resident jobs that I most wanted. Of course, it was not the only reason but I am fairly sure that it did play a part. I had to accept the fact that I was a failure as a doctor and that was appallingly difficult. I think that I had realized many years previously, perhaps before I could walk or talk, that I was a failure in the emotional world! I now had to accept that I was also a failure in the academic world and the adult world of work. Being clever had probably been my only worth in my own eyes and it was crippling to discover that my value had now gone. Life seemed hopeless. They were dark times and I did not know any way of showing my intense distress other than denying it and this meant that no help was available to me.

After many attempts and failures at work and periods of depression and exhaustion, however, I started training as an assistant in a general practice in a rural area south of Cambridge. In those days, unlike present times, this suggested failure as viewed from the hospital doctor's point of view. But for me it meant that I could use all my practical and clinical knowledge away from the pressures of hospital work. In those days general practice was incredibly varied, practical and often an adventure. My son is now working as a veterinary surgeon in a remote area in the Scottish Highlands and often I realize that my work then was more like his work now as a vet than a contemporary general practitioner's work. Home delivery of babies was the norm. There was a flying squad that could come and deal with an emergency but sometimes the crisis had to be sorted out before the squad had time to travel from Cambridge. Delivering a gypsy's baby by candlelight in a traditional wooden caravan with all the family around and one of the older women looking on and offering advice about the management of the delivery was not an isolated occurrence. I thrived on all this practical work and my health improved and my energy increased. Life seemed to have some meaning again and in many ways each day I felt that I was needed.

There were still times, however, when I looked back privately on all the failures behind me. I have written in some detail about these years because I now believe that the problems of those years had a lot to do with the further development and progress of MS. The conflict between my ideas of success and failure and their intimate connection with worth and lack of worth were resolved at that time by a greed to be needed. I think that it has been a greater understanding of this conflict that has contributed to my recovery since my severe relapse nearly two years before rewriting this book.

In my student days I had had many friends of both sexes but after I had failed and been 'condemned' to leave the hospital world I became more solitary. Knowing in my core that I was unlovable (I am sure that I did not see it as clearly as this at that time more than thirty years ago) my emotional survival rested on two pillars. One was academic success and that had collapsed with my left leg and the other was on being needed. The more I was needed by as many people as possible the greater my worth in my own eyes. Perhaps medicine and other caring professions are overstocked with those in desperate need of being needed and I was certainly one of them!

As my work progressed and my much shaken security increased, I began to make some new friends and one was John, whom I later married. We settled in the same area where I had been working and remained there for the next twenty years. My husband did not want me to go on working and I experienced a sense of loss. In due course we had three children and at the time I seemed remarkably well. I thrived during the pregnancies, had very easy labours and deliveries and few difficulties in breast feeding the babies. I became an 'earth' mother and was surprised at how much I enjoyed being at home with very small children. I certainly knew that I was very much needed during those years!

5

After the diagnosis of MS I looked back at this time and realized that I did have periods of ill-health which might have been caused by MS. After the birth of our second baby I developed double vision. It was a nuisance but there was little time to read or sew and so it caused me little hardship. I went to an oculist about it and she thought it was probably due to fatigue and that with sufficient rest it would clear up. Fatigue seemed a reasonable diagnosis because the first two babies were born only twenty months apart and life at that time was physically exhausting. The oculist was right and the vision got better after about three months.

Before and after the birth of our third child I had a weak left hand and a feeling of heaviness in both legs which made walking difficult. This pregnancy started less than a year after the birth of the second baby and during this time I put on a lot of weight, so feelings of heaviness seemed reasonable. Rest was almost impossible because of the amount of totally necessary work. I staggered through the pregnancy and some months after the birth of our younger daughter my legs felt better and my left hand returned to normal.

My husband was considerably older than I and by 1969 when the children were ten, eight and seven years old he was beginning to think about retirement. We were already having holidays in the north of Scotland. John's paternal grandmother had come from Caithness in the north-east of Scotland and he had the expatriate Scot's strong desire to return to an area where he felt his roots to be. We started looking for a cottage or land where we could make a holiday home and in due course a retirement home. Although I had no desire to leave East Anglia where I had come to feel I belonged I realized that John had no such feelings and that it would be better for the whole family if he could feel more tranquil. I could not have known at that time how wrong I was but perhaps the difficulties of the coming years would have occurred whether we had moved or not.

We found land overlooking one of the most beautiful harbours in the north-east of Scotland and built a house on the ruins of four cottages. Every window had a superb view over the Moray Firth or the harbour and a waterfall. We had looked at the local high school before the building started and at that time it seemed very good. Before our move north the children were all at private schools in Cambridge and the thought of the expense of continued private education after my husband's retirement was daunting. We both believed that they might fare better with a state secondary education in Scotland rather than in England. We also inquired about part-time work for me, and although there would be none at the time of our removal north there would probably be some after a year.

After the building of the house started in 1969 I had a hysterectomy and following this another period of weakness in both legs and my right arm. At that time I was working full-time and I managed to keep going for a year doing my own work, extra work during another doctor's study leave and looking after the children and house. Characteristically I seemed to be coping and coping well but it was only for a limited time. I became increasingly fatigued and eventually had to ask for time off work. At that time I was so exhausted and depressed that I was sent to a psychiatrist. I did not have any physical examination but was admitted to a nursing home for psychiatric treatment. I remember that I was so tired that I spent the first week asleep. I commented that it seemed like a physical illness but was reassured that depression has that effect. It is extraordinary that there is always this clear-cut distinction between what is mental illness and what is physical illness. There is also a distinction between acceptable physical illness and unacceptable mental illness.

We had our usual holiday in the north of Scotland in the summer of 1970 and I was then recovering from my fatigue. I can remember now, but did not draw attention to it at the time, that I had great difficulty walking on uneven ground and down cliff paths. I was embarrassed because I fell over frequently for no apparent reason.

John planned to retire the following year and I knew that there would be no regular part-time medical job for me during that first year. Leaving the south of England for me was like retiring because there were so many leaving parties and presents. All my friends and relatives who had always lived in the south-east or south-west of England thought we were crazy to be moving so far away and there were many times during that last year when I secretly shared their doubts. If I had known then that John would not retire until five years after that move and of all the other problems that would occur in the years ahead I should have tried to prevent the move. But now, fifteen years later, I can look back and see the pattern more clearly and do not regret the eight years spent in the Highlands of Scotland.

During 1973 I wrote my first book and this was some help during that first long, dark winter living in an isolated house with three children, finding it difficult to settle down. The local high school had by that time become comprehensive and the standards of education changed a great deal. Seeing the Northern Lights was beautiful and exciting and some compensation for the life and friends left behind in the south. There were many times during those early months when I had to remind myself how difficult it had been to get our small grand piano down the steep cliff path to our house and how impossible it would be to get it up again. But if some generous benefactor had offered me a move south I am sure that I would have accepted and abandoned the piano! But no such offer was forthcoming and we all had to learn to live in a different world in a different way.

My health in those early years in Scotland was good. Gradually I did some medical work on an irregular basis and a lot of journalism. The children adapted in some part to their new life and in restrospect I can feel fairly sure that it was easier for our son than our daughters. During that first year John accepted the chairmanship of his firm and all thought of imminent retirement vanished.

In 1975 I went to East Africa with John on a working visit. It was an interesting and exciting time and I thoroughly enjoyed being involved in his business interests there. We spent a lot of time looking at the sisal estates and inspecting some of the low-level waste-disposal areas where mosquitoes abounded. We were bitten many times but were both conscientious in taking our malarial preventatives and therefore were not worried. We returned home just before Christmas. Twelve days after our return I had a sudden attack of fever and was poorly for about twenty-four hours. The same thing happened again after a similar interval. This time I went to our doctor and suggested that I might possibly have malaria. It seemed a most unlikely diagnosis to be made in Caithness in the cold and dark of mid-winter. However, I was admitted to the hospital in Inverness, the diagnosis was confirmed and I returned home with bottles of pills.

That, I thought, should have been the end of the matter and I ought to be feeling better. But, alas, I was not feeling better and continued to feel exhausted and very low. My shoulders ached and my left hand was remarkably clumsy. 'That hand' kept dropping things and I felt increasingly angry with it. Eventually I went to see the consultant physician in Wick. By that time I was having some difficulty in walking and his examination showed abnormalities in my nervous system. At that time all the abnormalities were on my left side and he said that a brain tumour had to be ruled out. I went back to Inverness for the non-invasive tests including a brain scan and was then admitted to our local hospital for the invasive test, a lumbar puncture.

After all the tests were completed the consultant physician told me that I must now consider that the diagnosis was multiple sclerosis. He did say that a diagnosis at my age – I was then forty-nine years old – did not usually mean a rapidly serious outcome but a slow deterioration. The idea of a slow but inevitable deterioration, although it did not conjure up pictures of being in a wheelchair within the next few months, was certainly a devastating threat and was really too upsetting to think or talk about seriously. I was then, in effect, a single parent bringing up three teenagers far from old friends and in what inevitably remained an alien culture.

He told me about the positive things I could do and the first was to lose weight. I had gained an enormous amount of weight over the years since our move and in February tipped the scales at 13½ stone. Few of my clothes still fitted me and my shape, weak leg and clumsy hand all added to my dislike, possibly hatred, for my own body. He told me about avoiding 'hard' fats and taking instead supplements of sunflower seed oil. The diet seemed to be the only available bit of magic at that moment. After I had seen the dietician and been given a low calorie and low-fat diet I pitched into it quite fanatically as though my life depended on it. I saw it as something positive and constructive to do. But I am sure now, eleven years later, that the children saw my devotion to 'my diet' as stupid and an unwelcome intrusion into our family life. The diagnosis of MS and that diet became the pillars of my life.

I think that at the time of the diagnosis I intended to go on working as though nothing had happened, but, while suffering from a severe post-lumbar puncture headache, I collided on a bend in a narrow road with a parked van. It was probably not entirely my fault but at that moment I was quite prepared to make a statement to the police and confess to anything at all. My opinion of myself was so low that my own battered car and a damaged van could make little difference. The postman was not in the van and I was much shaken but not otherwise injured. The police took me to the hospital and the consultant physician ran me home in his car. Our general practitioner came down to see me and while he was there took the children into the kitchen and told them I had MS. To this day I have no idea what he or they said or really what the diagnosis meant to them. I could not ask them then and would not ask them now. I am quite certain that it was not helpful to them or to me at the time or in the years to follow. The diagnosis was impossible for me to understand and I suspect for them it was equally meaningless. Somehow we were all silenced. I was left with an unspeakable threat to my future and they were left with a mother who was concentrating on her own survival and pinning all her hopes on an incredibly restricted diet and a bottle of sunflower seed oil which she slurped down every morning rapidly followed by an orange. What a picture of family life!

My husband came home very rarely during that miserable year. From my point of view it seemed an appalling rejection and most unfair. But from his angle it must have seemed a ridiculous pursuit to travel seven hundred miles north of London, which was expensive and time-consuming, to go to a family which was unhappy and a wife who was shut up in herself and obsessed with her body's weakness and her diet. There is no doubt that the diagnosis drove us farther apart than the actual physical distance which separated us. I needed someone who could be a support to me and to whom I could talk about my fears and anxieties. He was not that sort of person and was unable to respond to my needs; and looking back I can see more clearly the inevitability of our increasing depth of separation. I felt a victim of the disease and of a rejecting husband and increasingly isolated inside my own treacherous body.

I stayed at home for about two months after the car crash and had a course of ACTH injections. At the time they seemed to help but I am not sure whether the improvement was due to the injections, the rest or the diet. Those weeks at home were a respite between the months of utter fatigue which preceded them and those of near despair which followed them. Perhaps I was numb from the diagnosis and the steroids may have given me some sort of 'high'. For three weeks my right hand was too shaky for me to write and I found that very disturbing; luckily it passed.

The diagnosis of MS meant for me, as it does for many and possibly the majority of people, a sentence of near-death. I should become paralysed inevitably, end up in a wheelchair, be incontinent and almost totally dependent on other people. I was living far away from old friends and relatives and was almost solely responsible for bringing up three teenage children. Part of me was strangely relieved that there was something physically wrong and that my weak limbs and devastating fatigue were not just 'all in the mind'; but another part of me was shocked and terrified that this awful thing could have happened to me. It really was one of those things that only happens to other people, like being struck by lightning or hit by a train on a level crossing.

At that time I did not know about benign forms of MS or that only one out of five people with MS actually ever needs a wheelchair. As a medical student I had learnt about and seen severe cases of MS and I am not at all sure that in the late 1940s when I trained that the benign disease had been recognized.

The curious sense of relief that it was a real physical disease was great and it meant that I now had an acceptable reason for feeling so tired and unwell. The alternative in the past was some sort of neurosis and that was not acceptable and had to be battled with. Physical disease was OK and was clearly separated from mental disease which was not. A physician or a general practitioner or a neurologist was the sort of doctor who treated MS and that was respectable; but a psychiatrist treated mental illness and that was definitely not respectable. So it seemed important at that time and many times since, in fact until the past two years, that my disease had physical signs and symptoms and not just mental or emotional ones. Somehow if it had the label of MS it was commendable.

If this disease was physical I was inevitably its victim. I could not in any way be responsible for a physical disease. That was how I saw it in 1976 and much had to happen to me before I could change my ideas of this hard divide between physical and mental disease and to come to my present understanding of the blurring of the two.

If I was the victim of the disease I could either accept it totally and the inevitability of becoming crippled; or I could fight against it in a limited way but without any real hope of winning. I did know that in one sort of MS there were relapses and remissions but I had been told that late-onset MS progressed without remissions, but slowly. I made a sort of pact with some spiritual power, which I later feared was the devil, that I should not become helpless for ten years. I reckoned that should be sufficient time for the children to become independent. After that I decided I should be redundant and it would not matter so much if I were helpless. That bargain was to become a frightening threat and almost a reality ten years later. It is strange how a decade can seem so long when looked at from the beginning and so brief a time when looked back on from the end!

In 1976, during the months following the diagnosis, I gradually pieced together other incidents which had occurred before my visit to East Africa. I recalled that in March of 1975 I had done some locum work in the local children's hospital and had caught some sort of virus infection which had lasted about a month. After I got better I had aching shoulders and also found that my left hand was clumsy and inclined to shake. I had found this embarrassing particularly on Monday mornings when I used to help the gynaecological surgeon in the operating theatre. If I held a retractor in my left hand for more than about a minute it started to shake. I felt very upset because I thought it must look as though I was drinking excessive amounts of alcohol. I found various surreptitious ways of supporting my hand so that it did not shake. One Monday I had to go and give a baby an injection after the stint in theatre. I found it almost impossible to control the movements of my left hand and I felt anxious. After any strenuous effort with the hand it was quite impossible to do any fine movements with it for some hours. It had crossed my mind on one occasion that this clumsy shaking hand could be due to MS but I forgot about it almost immediately and never allowed the thought back into my mind. The aching shoulders, the heavy feelings in my arms and my clumsy left hand lasted all that year. I also realized during that time I had dropped a great number of things, which was unusual for me. It had grieved me when a new jar of expensive instant coffee crashed to the floor; after that I learned to hold things in my right hand.

It was also during those months in 1976 that I began to understand the feelings of being disabled. I was never so disabled that I could not walk; but sitting and lying were much easier. I realized that the feeling of disability had more to do with my mind's feelings about my body than the reality of my physical body. This feeling of being damaged was very real and I sometimes had fantasies about some sort of maggot destroying my nervous system. Of course, I knew that this was a fantasy but there were times when what was happening to me was more like a waking nightmare than real life.

Until that time my body had belonged to me and for the most part had been healthy. When I was pregnant my feelings about my body were so changed that I felt everybody else must see the difference although it was too soon for there to be any observable physical enlargement. In the same way my feelings about disability and the damage that had been done and was being done to my body and particularly my nervous system, made it seem that it must be apparent to an outsider, which was not in fact the case. I think that at that time my feelings went like this: I was damaged; I hated my body being damaged; it was obviously damaged in the sight of everybody and therefore everybody must hate my body as much as I did. I had become in some way an outcast and unlovable but at least deserving of pity.

My husband's absence during that year increased my feelings of disability and my own resulting devaluation. He had always liked things that were physically attractive but now I knew that my body had become physically repulsive and this feeling was made worse by his rejection. My self-loathing increased in proportion to what I then saw as his rejection of me. I would not at that time have described my feelings as angry, which I now recognize them to be, but rather as helpless and despairing.

My only hope of salvation seemed to be the diet, so I grasped at it feverishly. Looking back I realize that I was obsessed with it and made an exhibition of it. At the time I thought I was being quiet, self-controlled and not showing my anxiety. I feel sure now that my obsession with the diet made the children angry and increased my isolation.

A neurologist friend in Australia wanted me to see a colleague of his in London. At the time he first made this suggestion, the distance to London and the effort necessary made it seem impossible. It was many months before I managed this journey. I said that I would not cross the 'ord' which is the line of hills separating Caithness from Sutherland and the south, until I could do it under my own steam. This meant being able to drive the 120 miles to Inverness to catch the main-line train to London. That time arrived in the autumn of 1976. I went to see this neurologist feeling resigned and aware that nearly ten months of my ten years' mobility, for which I had bargained, had gone, but I left him walking 'on air'. Seeing him was a small miracle. What was his magic?

He is a neurologist of international fame with a particular interest and expertise in MS. He gave me a lot more information about the disease which I knew would be correct because of his quiet certainty. He took a full history of my illness, gave me a most thorough physical examination and agreed with the diagnosis of MS. The great difference that visiting him made to me was my increased understanding of the disease. He said with certainty that I did not have a late-onset disease which meant the slow and progressive deterioration I had been told to expect. He believed that I had started the disease in my early twenties and it was a benign form of MS with some relapses but long remissions. The problems in the past year were just part of a relapse and that I was likely to go on improving and that I should regain much of my previous stamina. The whole future seemed to change and I felt more optimistic than I had done for many months.

I shall never be able to express my gratitude adequately to this remarkable man with his quiet manner, great clinical expertise and total integrity. I continued to see him at six-monthly intervals for several years. He could always make wise suggestions about the management of current physical problems. At one time I found it very difficult to sit and type for more than about twenty minutes because the upper part of my back ached so badly. He told me that a novelist patient of his had had the same problem and had solved it by having the typewriter on a steeply sloped surface. At first I used a tray propped up on a pile of books but later had a more stable and permanent version made. It was so simple but effective and this was the beginning of my own changed attitude to problems. Many could be solved with a little clear and creative thinking followed by action. I was not then any sort of victim of a problem. It was a most valuable attitude in which to be initiated although I should not reap the full benefit until many years later.

I remember going to have lunch with a friend after that first visit to the neurologist with my body feeling lighter and more active than it had done for a long time. I think about this doctor when I hear of patients' encounters with neurologists from whom they get no help, because there is nothing to be done; and indeed with my own most recent contact with another neurologist which left me confused, angry and lacking in hope. I suppose that in the physical and orthodox medical sense there is nothing to do because MS remains an untreatable and incurable disease; but there is plenty to do in the sense of helping the patient to understand his disease, come to terms with his limitations and be realistic about the future.

One of my continuing problems was that my husband seldom came home and did not believe that I had any physical disease. The neurologist offered to see him and tell him about the benign sort of MS which I had so that he could understand it better. But he never went. Looking back I see that the diagnosis of MS became an ever-growing fence between us. I relied on it as an excuse for whatever I was unable to do and a reason for my recurrent fatigue and depression. He said that the diagnosis was just one more example of my mental instability and that I was using the disease as an unfair and dishonest weapon against him. There was some justice in this but I failed to see one crumb of truth in such allegations until eighteen months ago.

I stuck to my diet and lost three stone in two months. Although it did my morale good to be taking in clothes or shopping for those two sizes smaller, the speed of the loss was a severe blow to my body. My energy was less and my fatigue greater. When I went back to work after two months at home, and I was only doing a part-time job, I found the tiredness frightening. I could get through the first day of work but by the middle of the second day I was 'dropping' into a chair, finding it difficult to stand up again or drive a car.

One afternoon when I arrived home particularly tired I telephoned the welfare officer at the Multiple Sclerosis Society in London. She told me that fatigue was a common problem and that more people gave up work on account of fatigue than loss of mobility. I was much comforted and from that time tried to work half-days instead of full ones and have a rest in the afternoon. Some weeks, if I was particularly tired, I spent a whole day in bed. I avoided driving long distances or even making long journeys by train. I thought that I should never again be able to have holidays far from home because the travelling would be too tiring and that it would be difficult to keep on my rigid diet. I was fitter without all my fat but in other ways those years in the mid-1970s were restricting ones and I was not much use as a wife or mother.

In July 1978 my husband retired from his full-time job in London but remained on the company's board of directors and made frequent trips for business purposes. Early in 1978 before his official retirement he had a severe attack of backache, arrived in Inverness on the night sleeper extremely unwell and was admitted to the hospital there. He was not happy about the treatment he was getting there and after a week decided to come home. The pain in his back improved but he became emotional and frequently tearful. He did not want me out of his sight and this was totally out of character for him. I wondered if he was having some sort of depressive illness but there was no way in which he would have accepted medical help for a mental illness and therefore all I could do was to be with him and try to support him. He kept saying that as soon as he retired he would start caring for me and the children and that was now all he wanted. For me it began to look as though his retirement really could be the beginning of a different sort of relationship and the one that I had hoped the move to Caithness might start. But, sadly, other things happened and now I understand that his retirement was not the beginning of a new life together but the start of his dementia (Alzheimer's disease) which led to his death eight years later.

He went back to London a few weeks before he left work and when he finally 'moved into' our home in Caithness he was unable to settle and enjoy any of the pursuits to which he had been looking forward for so many years. It is so easy to indulge in the 'if onlys' and I can easily start wishing that I had done this or that or had not been impatient and lacking in understanding.

Later that year the two elder children started at university. That was the beginning of frightening and disrupting problems with money. I had never known what John earned and I had always paid for the children's education while they were at fee-paying schools, and after the move to Scotland had subsidized the housekeeping. But the problem of parental contributions to university grants now loomed on the horizon. I discovered that the children would only get the minimum grant although John kept saying how poor he was, how small his pension and that he was unable to make any contribution at all to the expenses of the children at university. I became more anxious, perplexed and depressed about the future. I should not at the time have said I was angry about John's attitude; but I am sure now that underneath I was very angry.

The following year, 1979, our younger daughter decided she would prefer to go away to boarding school and work for some A-level examinations. This could have been the time when John and I might settle down together; but this did not happen. It is so easy to look back, apportion blame and feel guilt, but I still do not understand all the stresses or the effects of his dementia, which were not to be apparent for another four years. And by that time many terrible things had happened which are too painful and too private to be written about. For the purpose of writing about MS and the stresses which I believe led to my relapse suffice it to say that by the beginning of 1981 I was on my own in Norfolk.

In those two years our younger daughter had a devastating accident and many months in and out of hospital, I had a breakdown and John decided that I was responsible for the difficulties he was having in settling down in Scotland to enjoy his retirement. He decided he no longer wanted to go on with the marriage but would prefer to go and live with a cousin. For me there were frightening months without a job, a home or money. But I have wondered recently if my own MS is not better when I have no choices to make. For the next few years it was a question of survival.

I managed to get work, a mortgage on a very small terrace house in the centre of Norwich and so was able to provide some sort of resting place for myself and children. My husband would not allow me or the children to know his address or telephone number. I thought at first that there would be some division of his financial assets and at one point I saw a solicitor but I realized that it was useless although in 1981 I did not know the reason why. I gave up any idea of financial help and decided it was better to keep all my energy for getting on with my own life; and I was indeed fortunate to make new friends as well as renew old friendships. At regular intervals I telephoned John's cousin, who had found him a flat very near her, to ask about him; she always said he was well and she obviously enjoyed having him near. Apart from that there was no contact at all and he never got in touch with me.

There was one meeting in 1983 when our son wanted both his parents at his graduation ceremony in Edinburgh. I felt apprehensive at first but in the end the day went without a hitch. I spent some time alone with John. He seemed so sure of his own poverty and obsessed about his persecutors who were always sending him improper demands for money that I felt sincerely sorry for him. I assured him that I would never join the ranks of the people demanding money from him.

I remember saying during those years to one of my female medical contemporaries who was wondering how much part-time medicine she would like to do, that I was fortunate because I did not have any choice. If I did not work I had no money and without money I would be unable to pay the mortgage and if I could not pay the mortgage there would be no roof over our heads. Perhaps MS really is better under such conditions. Certainly I remained in very good health and with good stamina for several years. As one of my daughters said after her return from a holiday abroad where they had run out of money, 'If you are hungry and have almost no money it is quite easy. You just go and buy as much bread as you can!'

I did not make any contact with the MS Society and did not talk about my own illness. Apart from my numb left foot, my clumsy left hand and my tendency to lose my balance, particularly in the dark, I was well and not obviously disabled. Looking back now at those first five years on my own, I was, perhaps for the first time since I qualified, harnessing a lot of my talents and achieving some sort of small success in the medical profession. I once joked that at the time when most women were thinking about retirement I had just got into my stride and was starting out on my career. Having experienced that sort of buoyancy and optimism, the disappointment seemed much greater when my legs gave way, stopped me working and eventually prevented me from returning to clinical work.

During 1985 I had to see John again because his mental condition was deteriorating and his cousin found that she could no longer cope. At first I was very worried about being involved but when I realized the severity of John's dementia I had no choice. He no longer knew who I was, he would not see his general practitioner and he would accept no help of any kind. He was wandering at night and eventually he had to be taken to a mental hospital compulsorily. I had to arrange Court of Protection help so that I was able to pay for him in a nursing home. During 1985 there were other demands from members of the family; and each in its own way was an additional and tiring demand.

In November 1985 I had difficulty getting up the stairs at work. I had always worked in an attic room in the Victorian house which was used as the family planning clinic. I could manage the flight to the first floor but the second flight to my consulting room was much steeper. Halfway up this flight my right leg seemed to buckle and I could get no further without hauling myself up using the banisters or using my hands on the stairs ahead. At first I was worried about the indignity of the situation and I went through various ploys to make sure that anybody else coming up was ahead of me. Normally there was a bell to summon the next patient or a nurse from the floor below but during that time the bell was often out of action. I have no idea what I thought the problem could be in my leg. This may seem strange but I know that the thought of MS did not enter my conscious mind.

The same problem started happening at home but I avoided going up the stairs as much as possible. When I carried a hot drink upstairs to bed at night I put the drink a few stairs ahead of me and then followed it up using two hands on the stair ahead. I went privately to a physiotherapist to ask her to do something about the leg. She used various treatments but the leg got no better. I realize while writing that 'the leg' was no longer 'my leg' or part of my body and I believe this was how I saw the problem at that time. 'The leg' was letting me down literally as well as metaphorically and was therefore no longer an acceptable part of me.

Eventually, a week before Christmas, I realized that the struggle was too great, the left leg was getting as weak as the right and that I could no longer work. I fully accepted the relationship between the stresses that I was living with and weakness of my legs, but at that moment I believed this was a psychiatric illness and that the weakness was all in the mind. It had to be either mind or body and I was sure at this point it was mind.

In 1981 the Health Authority had arranged for me to see a neurologist before I started work. He had confirmed the clinical diagnosis of MS but thought that I was fit enough to do a part-time job. For me, in December 1985, having weak legs was a crisis and I expected to be seen instantly if anybody thought that this was physical illness. I was still unable to accept that this really was an exacerbation of MS. The neurologist was busy and I was given an appointment in January. I felt desperate and he finally saw me one evening in out-patients a day or so before Christmas. The whole thing seemed a disaster for which I wanted instant help. For him it was a run-of-the-mill relapse in chronic MS. He confirmed it was a relapse and showed more involvement of various parts of the spinal cord. He paid me the compliment of talking in medical terms which at that moment I was incapable of understanding. All I wanted was something, just about anything, to make me better. I could not possibly have an incurable and progressive disease because I needed good health! What remarkable arrogance on my part, but I do believe that was how I felt.

He did not believe in ACTH, diet or any other way of positive managment; but he did send me for some blood tests because, as he observed, members of the medical profession could have bizarre illnesses. I felt that some disease other than MS was my only hope. There still might be a treatment which could make me better. Because of Christmas, the results would not be available for a while. But when should I be able to get back to work? His reply was like a death sentence. 'I have no idea when you will get back to work again – or even if you will be able to.' I babbled stupidly about having to get back to work because I had a mortgage to pay and nobody to help me. It was a desolate moment and I was left almost without hope. I could see no way of managing again if this was not an illness that could be treated and put right. At that moment the choice seemed to be getting back to work and paying the mortgage or not getting back to work and becoming homeless.

I came home that evening quietly desperate and unable to see any way through the apparently insuperable problem. Deep down I think that I was aware that I needed and even wanted help in sorting out all the problems that I had managed to accumulate in the previous year or so but I was too angry to let my needs be known. All I wanted at a superficial level was somebody to, at least, make my MS better and then I thought that I should be able to cope with the rest. I felt so physically exhausted, and had so much muscle cramp and weakness, particularly in my thighs, that it seemed quite unreasonable that there was not somewhere some sort of treatment that would make this terrible disease better. I knew intellectually that if it was MS there was nothing much that anybody could do; but I just hoped desperately that it was something else that would be treatable.

But it *was* MS and over the next two years I had to learn gradually and painfully that 'the MS' could not be separated from 'me' and that any sort of recovery was impossible without the full involvement of me. There were many problems I had to face and resolve and much thinking, learning and understanding to be done before there was any relief from my symptoms. The first enormous lesson I had to relearn was to accept help. I needed it, not only because I had weak legs and could not drive a car or get to the shops, but because I was sick in many ways and at many levels. I began to see that I could not separate my muscle weakness from my many other problems. But this understanding of my sickness was slow and difficult and could only have happened with the help of many and different people and influences.

During the previous five years I had been going it alone and surviving against all odds; now I was dependent. For six weeks I was unable to drive and either had to stay at home or accept lifts. I accepted lifts, although I felt some embarrassment at being a parcel that might need to be moved from car to car. My friends were long-suffering and continued to offer help. One particularly good friend did my shopping on Saturday mornings but he had to accept lunch from me before I could accept help from him. How pathetic I was to believe that I could always be the helper and never the helped and always the carer and never the cared-for.

The difference I felt in my mind and heart between caring and being cared for was so profound that to cross the divide had been emotionally unthinkable. Caring was something I could control, that I could actually learn to do better, was mostly successful and, up to a certain point, the results could be anticipated. There was always the great reward, for me, of being needed. That kept up my value. To be cared for was not just the opposite but was a threatening purgatory. It meant total insecurity and confusion. If I could not be needed I was of no value. Therefore to join the ranks of the needy was a sort of emotional suicide and there was no middle ground between being needed and joining the ranks of the needy. It meant total loss.

I was losing all control over myself and my life. It meant total insecurity and becoming the victim not only of MS but of the powerful helpers because the medical profession in the guise of the neurologist had already rejected me. They had not been able to provide instant magic for me at the moment I wanted it so that I could get back to my chaotic life. I was not only being needed by my patients but also by my husband, my mother and other members of my family. What value I must have to be so needed: and what a fall from that height to being old, sick, out of work and out of control. I saw the difference at that time as the divide between some sort of heaven and a very definite hell. The two were irreconcilable.

I was in danger of becoming a victim and at that time I was only dimly aware of the enormous anger inside this victim. The anger had to be kept under wraps because its potential could be so dangerous. It was a sort of mini-volcano which had to be kept out of sight and understanding at all times and hidden from all people including the owner. For me the understanding and acceptance of this frightening anger within me was the beginning of healing. It was a long, demanding, painful and dangerous path; and it could have been simpler and superficially safer to have remained sick and progressively sicker and more disabled. I do not know that my path is applicable to anybody else and I am certainly not claiming it as a new treatment for MS, but perhaps another step in the understanding of this strange disease and possibly a guide to any people with MS who want to find their own path back to some sort of health.

My helpers have been many and varied and I do not believe there is a value for others with MS of writing in detail about each one. I think that the important thing has been that I have accepted help knowing that I needed it. Also, I have been the chooser of help and have never been in the position of having to accept help which I have not chosen or wanted. Being in control of the help has been important for me. To have become part of a mobilization programme or similar project might have been of help in the short term but I do not believe it would have been of great value in the long term.

My physical health has improved remarkably during the past two years and in the third part of this book I shall attempt to describe some of the moments which, for me, have been landmarks and which might spark off ideas for other people with MS and their helpers. I am sure that the way of help is unique for each person and I do not believe that the ways in which I have been helped and healed could be a blueprint for anybody else because that would deny the uniqueness of the individual. My own experiences during this time have stressed for me the importance of self-understanding rather than acceptance of some formula from outside, whether it is diet, rest, exercise or any other suggested management of the disease. I can offer only a menu which in the second part of this book will be the medically accepted (or disputed) items and in the third part will be those which I have found helpful but are very much my own ideas and experiences.

Part Two

Chapter 2   MS – the disease

Multiple sclerosis is a relatively 'new' disease and was first described by Jean-Martin Charcot, a French neurologist, in 1868. Charcot started working at the Salpetrière Hospital in Paris in 1862 and making careful clinical observations on all the long-stay patients there. From these observations he started to classify groups of signs and symptoms and made a number of clinical diagnoses. He was able to check his clinical diagnoses by post-mortem examinations after a patient's death. One of the diagnoses he made was MS, or disseminated sclerosis (*sclerose en plaques*) as it was first known, but in this hospital he was seeing and describing the severe and terminal cases of the disease. In 1868 he described the trio of symptoms of scanning speech, nystagmus and an intention tremor which became known as Charcot's triad and which do occur in severe MS. During the 1940s and 1950s, in London, I was still taught about Charcot's triad as diagnostic of MS. Benign MS, although it had already been described remained totally unknown to me. I remained ignorant of this type of MS until I saw a neurologist in 1976. This conception of MS as a very severe disease goes on and means unnecessary fears for a patient and his family and friends when a diagnosis of MS is made. The great anxiety surrounding the disease can lead to deceptions and evasions between doctors and patients. Only when a more realistic understanding of MS as a disease, which for the majority of people will have a benign course, is possible will communications about it become more honest.

Although a great deal of research has been done on the disease, particularly in the past twenty years, the cause of MS is not yet known but there are many possibilities. Ways of preventing and treating the disease also remain problematic without any definite answers.

The number of people in a community who get MS depends on the geographical position of that community. Near the equator the incidence is very low and it increases as one moves farther from the equator. There is more MS in the USA and Canada than there is South America and more in Tasmania than in Northern Queensland and more in the South Island of New Zealand than North Island; and more in Orkney and Shetland than in the south of England. This 'latitude' effect may be modified by the ethnic-genetic factors of the inhabitants. In Wellington, New Zealand, there is a relatively large amount of MS in those of European origin but it is a rare disease in the Maori population. Similarly, although Japan resembles New Zealand in latitude and climate, MS is uncommon in the Japanese.

It may vary from one part of a country to another. This happens in Norway where it is lower in coastal areas and higher in inland areas. It also happens in the United Kingdom where the disease is most common in Caithness and the Orkney and Shetland Islands. The incidence of MS in the Faroe Islands, which are north-west of the Shetland Islands is of particular interest. Before the Second World War there had been only two reported cases. Between 1940 and 1945 the Islands were occupied by British, mainly Scottish troops and between 1943 and 1960 there were twenty-three reported cases of MS in native Faroese people. After 1970 there was only one reported case. This sudden start and equally sudden disappearance does look as though there was possibly some sort of infection connected with the spread of the disease.

You retain the likelihood of developing MS depending on the area where you lived before the age of sixteen years. If you move from a high-risk to a low-risk area before that age your chances will change to low risk, but if you move after the age of sixteen you will keep the chances of a high-risk area.

European Mediterranean communities, who not only live in a warmer climate but who are predominantly Roman Catholics and are oil-eating and wine-drinking, have less chance of getting MS than their more northern neighbours who are more likely to be Protestant, fat-eating and beer or wine-drinking. Oil is a fat which is fluid at room temperature while fat is solid. The more passive Roman Catholics of southern Europe may be less tense, driving, compulsive characters than their northern neighbours.

What is the cause of MS?

In spite of the research done and many theories there are still no clear facts about what causes MS. It is almost certain that the cause is multifactorial. If I stand a full cup of coffee on my desk it does not automatically spill over; but if I stand it on a pile of papers it is more likely to spill; and if the desk has a fault in one of its feet the coffee is much more likely to spill because of the combination of risks. You do not get MS because you grew up in Orkney; but if you did and have several other 'risk' factors you are much more likely to get it than if you grew up in the south of France. There is also a difference between factors which cause something and those which are associated with the same thing. There is less MS in Italy, which is predominantly a Roman Catholic country and more in Orkney where most people will be members of the Church of Scotland. But nobody believes that attendance at a Church of Scotland service will cause MS; or becoming Roman Catholic will prevent you getting MS. These are factors which are associated with the community where MS has a high or a low incidence. There are probably some predisposing factors such as where you live, what you eat and what your genetic make-up is and then precipitating factors which could possibly be a virus infection or some sort of stress. But, I emphasize that none of this is yet known definitely.

The virus theory

The arrival of MS in the Faroe islands and its subsequent disappearance would favour some sort of infection theory. However, it is not a straightforward infection and it is not infectious from one person to another like the common cold. It could be due to a virus which causes an initial recognizable infection such as measles and then hangs around in the body for many years before the first signs of MS appear. In some people with MS increased levels of antibody to measles are present in the cerebro-spinal fluid, which is the fluid surrounding the brain and spinal cord, and the blood. Normally, after an infection is over, the antibody levels fall. At one time it was thought that it was those who got measles at a relatively late age who were at this sort of risk. But nobody believes that measles causes MS; only that the measles or some other virus might have something to do with it.

There are viruses that are known to hang around in the body for many years before causing further damage. The herpes simplex virus infects the majority of children in the UK before the age of five years and then stays quietly hidden in the body. But it can erupt and cause cold sores at a time when the person is under stress or exposed to an unusual amount of sunlight. The virus which causes chicken-pox similarly lies dormant and later, often when the person is under some emotional strain or suffering from another illness, causes shingles. More recently it has been discovered that the AIDS virus, after an initial infection, stays in the body and at a later time becomes active. The big difference between the AIDS virus and any possible connection between MS and a virus is that the person with AIDS is infectious from the time of infection and this is definitely not so in MS. The enormous amount of research being done world-wide on the AIDS virus could possibly have some benefit for understanding the causes of MS.

It is almost certain that any virus connected with MS does not act directly on the nervous system but has an effect on the body that makes it take action against its own nervous system. Normally the human body recognizes its own cells and when fighting a disease can recognize the difference between invaders and the home team; but in some diseases this recognition does not occur and the body turns against itself. Diseases caused in this way are called auto-immune diseases and include such diseases as Hashimoto's thyroiditis, one sort of disease of the thyroid, and possibly diabetes and some types of arthritis. Drugs which have been used for the treatment of MS, such as ACTH, damp down this self-destructive, almost 'suicidal' sort of behaviour by the body.

In the past there have been other suggestions for connecting MS with some sort of infection. These include 'scrapie' in sheep, a neurological disease spread by a virus. It has a high incidence in Orkney and it was suggested that the virus that caused this disease in sheep might be passed to man and be responsible for MS. This was not substantiated by further observation. It was also suggested that the virus that caused neurological diseases in dogs, such as distemper, could be passed to humans and cause MS; but again this idea did not stand up to further investigation.

Genetic factors and MS

Although it appears probable tht MS is in some way related to viral infection it must be stressed that it cannot be passed from one person to another like influenza. Similarly, although it is known that relatives of people with MS have an increased chance of developing the disease, MS is not inherited in an understandable way as it is in diseases such as cystic fibrosis or Huntington's chorea. It seems that what you can inherit is an increased susceptibility to the disease. About 10–15 per cent of people with MS have a member of the family also affected. Perhaps it is important to stress that 85–90 per cent do not have any relative affected. Canadian studies have shown that it is more common for identical twins to develop MS than fraternal twins who have the same risk as any other non-twin siblings. Again, it must be stressed that less than a third of identical twins do develop MS when the other twin has the disease. This shows that other factors must be at work apart from genetic ones because identical twins have identical genes.

There also seems to be some sort of genetic protection against the disease as shown by the low incidence of the disease in certain ethnic groups such as the Japanese, Maoris, Eskimos, the black population of Africa, Australian Aborigines and Indians.

It is suggested that the human leucocyte antigen (HLA) system of the body is the one associated with the ethnic and geographical distribution of MS. This system is one of closely linked genes on chromosome 6 and is responsible for controlling the manufacture in the body of many antigens and the control of immunity. This HLA system is inherited as a single set of genes from each parent, and possession of certain HLA types causes an increased susceptibility to certain diseases. These diseases include ankylosing spondylitis, thyroiditis, psoriasis and coeliac disease. There is a frequent association between particular types of HLA antigen and the development of MS. About 60 per cent of MS patients have a particular group of HLA antigens compared with 20 per cent in the population at large. These antigens are rare in the ethnic groups where MS is an uncommon disease.

Although they are not necessary for the development of MS, these antigens do make the individual who has them more susceptible to development of the disease. There may be an agent, common in nature, causing the disease; whether or nor MS develops is largely determined by the age of the person when exposure occurs and the HLA make-up of the person. The disease can then remain sub-clinical and in one-third of patients arrest or prolonged remission occurs after the initial symptoms. However, in the people who have a genetically-determined inability to make an adequate immunological response, the classic disease of MS develops with its characteristic progress of relapses and remissions.

What is the connection between MS and diet?

An American neurologist, Swank, wrote in 1950 about a connection between MS and different types of fat in the diet, using the incidence of MS in Norway to support his hypothesis. In the coastal areas of Norway where oil is eaten the incidence of MS is lower than inland areas where fat is eaten. He advised a diet rich in polyunsaturated fat and this has been adoped in many areas in the management of MS. The intake of fat in MS is interesting because the myelin sheath which surrounds the nerves, and is the part destroyed in MS, is made of fat, and it was suggested by Dick in 1976 that demyelination was more likely in the presence of saturated fat than in the presence of unsaturated fat.

It is also known that there are some fatty acids, called essential fatty acids (EFAs), which cannot be manufactured in the body. It has been suggested that people who have MS may have low levels of linoleic acid, one of the EFAs; this is the reason for using evening primrose oil.

Other factors connected with MS

MS is more common in women of all ages than men, but female deaths from MS peak after the menopause: it has been suggested that there is possibly a hormonal factor in the development of MS.

As paralytic polio used to be, MS is commoner in higher socio-economic classes as described by the Registrar-General. It is possible that those in lower socio-economic classes are exposed to more types of infection at a younger age because of lower standards of hygiene. In tropical countries, for example, where drinking water is likely to be impure, many viruses such as that causing polio will be widely spread and a natural immunity may develop early in life. This is only a theory and like so many things about MS has not been proved.

What happens to the nervous system in MS?

The individual patches of disease in MS are in the brain and spinal cord. They are not in the nerves of the head, body, arms or legs, where the symptoms may occur. (Symptoms are those things of which a person complains such as tingling in an arm or weakness in a leg. Signs are those things which a doctor finds during an examination.) Each nerve has a central bundle of nerve fibres and is surrounded by a myelin sheath. This sheath is made up of mostly polyunsaturated fatty material. In MS this sheath is damaged, and under the microscope the reaction looks like inflammation. The damage usually starts near a small vein and it has been suggested that whatever causes the damage arrives via the blood. This would fit in with either a viral or auto-immune cause.

At the time of the breakdown of the nerve sheath there is some swelling in the nerve and in the surrounding parts and an increase in the number of white corpuscles in the area. After this initial reaction, during which there is a varying amount of interference with the action of the nerve affected, the destructive process stops and the swelling goes. It was said that the nerve sheath could not recover, but it is now believed that limited recovery is possible. The signs of damage to the nerve itself often disappear completely although they may reappear during a relapse.

The MS lesions seem to appear on the parts of the brain and spinal cord exposed to cerebro-spinal fluid (CSF). This fluid circulates through the ventricles, which are small spaces within the brain, and around the brain and spinal cord. The swelling caused by the reaction in MS may be particularly important at places where nerves pass through narrow bony canals in the skull; and this is true of the optic nerve which is necessary for vision. More damage will be done if the swelling at these sites continues for any length of time.

How does MS start?

The onset of MS may be so insignificant that a doctor is not consulted and the diagnosis is often only made in retrospect after a further incident or incidents. MS, on the other hand, can start more dramatically and the person be unmistakably ill. The eventual outcome does not depend on the acuteness of the onset. The so-called 'late onset' MS which seems to start in the forties or fifties is possibly not a different type of illness but the manifestation of a relatively benign type of MS in which there have already been a number of minor episodes. It is quite impossible to give a description of typical MS because the disease is characterized by its infinite variability.

The first symptoms may be in the eyes, with blurring of vision in one or both eyes and possibly some pain. This is due to a lesion in the optic nerve and if the patient is examined at this time with a light shone into his eye with an ophthalmoscope, a whitening may be seen of the optic disc at the back of the eye. This disc is the end of the optic nerve and if the lesion is just behind the disc it may be possible to see that the disc is swollen. At this time vision may not only be blurred but there may be an absent patch in the middle of the normal field of sight. Diplopia or double vision may be the first symptom of MS. Neither of these eye problems, although suggestive of MS, makes the diagnosis a certainty and it seems to me quite reasonable, even if the diagnosis is suspected at this stage, that it should not always be disclosed. There may well be a period of many years before any other symptoms appear and in the absence of any proven cure or method of preventing a relapse, a doctor could be well advised to keep his suspicions to himself.

Another early symptom may be weakness or altered sensation in one or more limbs, most commonly a leg. The weakness may be felt as a heaviness and difficulty in lifting a foot off the floor. The use of a hand

34

may be so upset that it can be described as a 'clumsy' hand. The changes in sensation can be tingling or a feeling of a tight band, numbness or feelings of cold. If the limbs are examined at this stage there may be little to find and the amount of weakness which can be demonstrated on examination is often less than the patient feels. This is a characteristic of the disease and not a proof that the patient is 'putting it on'. The tendon reflexes in the affected limb or limbs may be slightly increased and there may be loss of a sense of touch and vibration as shown by putting a tuning fork on a bony area at the end of a limb. Sometimes, in apparently more severe forms of MS, there is an early loss of balance and severe giddiness and vomiting.

The first symptoms can disappear completely although on examination some signs of disease remain. Sometimes it is as many as twenty years before there are further symptoms; on the other hand, there may be more symptoms after only a few months. It is believed that the longer the interval between the first and subsequent symptoms, the better the outlook. This is very difficult to estimate because the first symptoms may have occurred many years before the diagnosis of MS and been unnoticed.

Occasionally, a patient has shown the early symptoms of MS and then no further symptoms at any time. One or two of those people who complained of mild symptoms suggestive of MS and who did not develop any further symptoms later died of a disease completely unrelated to MS. When the brain and spinal cord were examined after death the characteristic lesions of MS were found. This suggests that it is possible for an indefinitely long remission to occur and during life it may look as though the disease is cured. For this reason it is probably a mistake to discuss the diagnosis at the first occurrence of suggestive symptoms.

There are frequently bladder symptoms. These can be relatively mild, such as urgency, which is having to pass urine as soon as one feels the need; or symptoms can be more severe and eventually result in failure to control the passage of urine.

If and when symptoms do reappear they may be the original ones that come back or, more commonly, others are added. They can include unsteadiness in walking, a tremor or shake in either or both hands, changes of sensation in the body as well as the limbs, and often

35

muscle spasm and twitching in an affected leg. Pain is not usually a marked feature but muscle spasms can be very uncomfortable. At times there may be difficulties with speech.

Mental symptoms

MS euphoria is described as the failure of a person to realize the nature of the illness and has been described as a feature. I have not experienced euphoria or met any person with MS who has it. Depression is much more common and often out of proportion to the severity of the illness at the time. I believe now that this depresion has something to do with the onset of the disease and the times at which relapses occur. Depression and MS can both be illnesses which are characterized by a turning-in on oneself and also of denial of anger. Fatigue is a very common complaint and there is also a general loss of stamina in both physical and mental spheres. This loss of energy, the physical symptoms and the depression are common and are essential parts of MS.

I have had fears, and met others with MS who have shared them, about dementia. At one point I was foolish enough to look this up in a textbook and saw what was written about it. In theory it can happen late in the illness but the common complaints of loss of memory and poor concentration are, I believe, connected with depression and are not heralds of early dementia. If you are preoccupied with the physical disease and fears about the present and future, you are tied up inside yourself and will not be as aware of the world outside. It is natural that if you are not able to concentrate on things going on around you that you will fail to remember many of them. Many of these mental problems will disappear as better physical health comes.

Chapter 3   Investigations and Diagnosis

Although the likelihood or probability of the diagnosis of MS can be made with some certainty during a person's life, the definitive diagnosis of MS can only be made with certainty in a post-mortem examination. All the lesions are locked away in the central nervous system (CNS) and their presence can never be proved completely during life; unfortunately at the present time there is no specific test for MS.

Diagnostic guides for a diagnosis of MS

In 1983 the Poser Committee accepted that there are always doubts about the diagnosis of MS and laid down guide-lines for diagnosing so-called 'definite' and 'probable' MS under the two categories of clinical and laboratory-supported evidence for the disease.

The Poser Committee Diagnostic Guides for MS

1 Clinically definite MS
   a Two attacks and clinical evidence of two separate lesions.
   b Two attacks, clinical evidence of one and paraclinical evidence of another separate lesion.

2 Laboratory-supported definite MS
   a Two attacks, either clinical or paraclinical evidence of one lesion and cerebro-spinal fluid (CSF) abnormalities.
   b One attack, clinical evidence of two separate lesions and CSF abnormalities.
   c One attack, clinical evidence of one and paraclinical evidence of another separate lesion, and CSF abnormalities.

3 Clinically probable MS
  a Two attacks and clinical evidence of one lesion.
  b One attack and clinical evidence of two separate lesions.
  c One attack, clinical evidence of one lesion and paraclinical evidence of another, separate lesion

4 Laboratory-supported probable MS
  a Two attacks and CSF abnormalities.

Note An 'attack' is the occurrence of a symptom or symptoms of neurological dysfunction which lasts for more than twenty-four hours.

Clinical diagnosis of MS

For a clinically definite diagnosis of MS there must 'ideally' be two attacks, with some clinical evidence of those attacks, in different parts of the CNS; each attack must have lasted at least twenty-four hours and the two attacks must be separated by at least a month. This will show that the disease is 'multiple' both in time and space. The symptoms which will support such a diagnosis have been described previously.

Investigations which may support the diagnosis

Investigations may be done for the following reasons;

1 Sometimes early symptoms of MS can look like other diseases not in the CNS and tests can show that there is disease in the CNS.

2 Tests may confirm that a disease that looks like MS clinically is MS.

3 At the start of the disease MS may look as though there is disease at only one site in the CNS. Certain tests may however show that there are lesions in other places in the CNS and so support the diagnosis of MS.

4 The symptoms that look like MS may occur in other diseases of the CNS; investigations may be necessary to rule out – or confirm – the presence of such a disease.

5 When clinical trials of a new treatment are being done, tests may be necessary to assess the value of the therapy and to avoid the occurrence of side-effects.

Some of these tests are made routinely in neurological practice, others are more restricted because of limited availability, or, because of limited clinical value at present, some tests are made only in research units. The following table summarizes the investigations routinely available, although nuclear magnetic resonance imaging (NMRI) is not yet widely available.

Table One

Investigation	Reason(s) for requesting investigation
Blood examination	To exclude other diseases, e.g. subacute combined degeneration of spinal cord due to vitamin B_{12} deficiency.
Lumbar puncture/CSF examination	To determine if changes characteristic of MS are present.
Electroencephalography (EEG)	Only indicated if patient has had a 'blackout' – to determine its nature.
Electrodiagnosis Evoked Potentials Visual (VEP) Brain Stem-Auditory (BAEP) Somato-Sensory (SSEP)	The detection of sub-clinical lesions in: optic nerves brain stem spinal cord-brain.
Radiology Metrizamide Myelography with Computerized Tomography Computerized Tomography of Brain (CT scan) Nuclear Magnetic Resonance Imaging (NMRI)	To detect sub-clinical lesions and to exclude other pathologies in spinal cord and brain.

Lumbar puncture and examination of CSF

In doubtful cases of MS, examination of the CSF may provide useful information because there will be abnormalities in 50 per cent of MS patients. One abnormality is the increased amount of protein and another the increased level of immuno-gamma globulin which supports the theory that MS may be in part an immunological type of disease.

The CSF is obtained by a lumbar puncture which, although a routine procedure for the neurologist, can be an alarming investigation for the patient. It is particularly frightening because it has to be done 'behind your back' and if you are very apprehensive the doctor doing it may order a mild sedative. The patient lies on his left side on the edge of a bed or operating table with his knees drawn up to his chest and supported by a nurse. A local anaesthetic is injected between the third and fourth lumbar vertebrae (just above the 'tail' bone) after the area has been cleaned with spirit. A fine bore needle is then inserted and after measuring the pressure of the CSF with a manometer a few millilitres are collected in test tubes for the pathologist to examine.

The procedure is similar when metrizamide myelography is done as part of the investigations. In this case it is usual for the lumbar puncture and removal of CSF to be done at the same time as the myelography and in the radiology department.

It is important for patients to be reassured that lumbar puncture and metrizamide myelography have no harmful effects on MS. Many patients have a headache after lumbar puncture but this can usually be prevented by the patient's staying flat in bed for a few hours after the investigation has been finished.

Electrodiagnosis

Advances in electronics have made it possible to measure the speed of the impulses travelling along a nerve; demyelination of a nerve, which occurs in MS, will slow down the travelling time of such impulses and this delay can actually be recorded. Such tests are called Visual Evoked Potential (VEP) responses. The tests are 'non-invasive', can be repeated frequently if necessary and are of no risk to the patient. The tests are of particular value in providing evidence of a latent lesion and so making a diagnosis more likely. For example, if a patient between the ages of twenty and forty, with no previous history of symptoms which could be MS, sees a doctor with a weak leg and a VEP shows that there has been demyelination in an optic nerve possibly having occurred some years ago, the diagnosis of MS is much more likely.

The test is most often done on the optic nerves because they are or have often been affected by demyelination during the course of MS. The patient sits in front of a board which is rather like a chess board. Electrodes are placed on the patient's head and all the patient has to do is sit and look at the board while the black and white squares alternate. The electrical response in the brain, caused by the patient's vision, is observed by the operator on a screen and printed out. This will show the slowing of the impulse through the nerve if it has been affected by demyelination; and this effect can last for years after the damage has been done by demyelination in MS. These tests can also be done on the auditory nerves, which are the ones involved in hearing, and on the peripheral nerves in the body and limbs. It must be stressed these tests are not absolutely specific for MS and positive results do occur in other diseases. Tests done on the optic and autitory nerves are more reliable than those done on peripheral nerves.

Neuroimaging

These tests for MS are advances in the diagnosis of demyelination in the brain and spinal cord: they can be used to show evidence of single or multiple lesions early in the course of MS but again are not specific tests for diagnosing MS. They include Computerized Axial Tomography (CT scanning) and nuclear magnetic resonance imaging (NMRI). The CT scan first became available in the 1970s and is a non-invasive test, does not cause any discomfort for the patient and can be used for in-patient or out-patient investigation. The CT scan is not a straightforward X-ray of the brain but can show changes of density in the brain and spinal cord by a computerized mathematical reconstruction. Areas of demyelination will show up as areas of lower density; a CT scan can eliminate the diagnosis of a cerebral tumour, which will show as an area of higher density, and can also be used to show the improvement in demyelination during treatment with steroids in an active phase of MS. The whole investigation using a CT scanner can be done in less than an hour. An intravenous injection may be given that will show the lesions more clearly. Theoretically the CT scanner has been displaced by the use of the Nuclear Magnetic Resonance Imager but CT scanners are at present more widely available.

Nuclear magnetic resonance imaging (NMRI) was first reported as a possible test for diagnosing MS in 1982. The technique is non-invasive, does not upset the patient and does no damage. It is useful because it can show plaques of MS in the brain, which may not be producing any symptoms at the time of the examination and which always have been 'silent' or symptom-free. It is not as useful for showing evidence of lesions in the spinal cord. The test works because demyelinated nerve tissue has lost much of its fat content which has been replaced by water and this change is picked up by the strong magnetic field from the radio waves used. The images are then picked up and recorded by an imager scanning the radio waves. Because it is not using ionizing radiation, as in X-rays, it is safer for repeated use. As with CT scanning the lesions shown could be due to diseases other than MS.

When NMRI was first used it was thought to be a very reliable way of diagnosing MS but it has now been realized that it may be too sensitive. The investigation could show evidence of lesions which never have and possibly never will cause a problem for the patient. NMRI should not be used for screening a patient after a first episode of optic neuritis because it may show further evidence of MS lesions and the likelihood or possibility of developing MS which may never occur. It also has limited availability because both the costs of buying the machines and running them are high.

Chapter 4   Treatment and Management of MS

There is at present no known cure for MS although many claims are and have been made for a 'new cure'. All such claims must be treated with great caution and it has been the doctor's difficult job to advise patients on which 'cures' could be tried, which might possibly be of help, and which would not have serious side-effects. It must be stressed that there is no known treatment which will take away MS, but some can be of benefit to patients and there are remedies for helping some symptoms.

The Randomized Controlled Trial

In a disease with so many normal variations in the symptoms and signs as well as the patient's feelings of fatigue or well-being, it is difficult to assess the benefits of any new treatment; but some attempt must be made to assess the possible benefits scientifically. The Randomized Controlled Trial (RCT) is used by the medical profession in an attempt to be objective. Two sets of people are chosen who are matched for age, sex, marital status and, in the case of MS, the activity or relative inactivity of the disease. They are then allocated, without their knowledge or the knowledge of the doctors controlling the trial, to a treatment group or a control group. To make the trial even more scientific, both groups are given identical-appearing capsules, pills or whatever is being tried. Obviously this cannot be done when an attempt is being made to show the value of a particular diet. Anyone would recognize a gluten-free diet.

Each person is examined at the beginning of the trial and again at the end. Their progress during the trial and any relapses or remissions are recorded. Only at the end will the doctors know who had the 'real' treatment and who had the 'imitation' or placebo treatment. In some trials, not only for MS, it has been found that as many people will improve with a placebo as with the drug undergoing a trial. Sometimes this can show the power that interest and suggestion can play in the relief of symptoms; but in MS it may also be evidence of a spontaneous remission which has occurred during the time of treatment and which has had nothing to do with the treatment. It is these normal fluctuations in the course of the disease that make any new treatment of MS so difficult to evaluate. It is also difficult to judge which patients to put into each group because the amount of disease clinically detectable in anyone may vary from day to day. Therefore, it is extremely difficult to compare 'like with like' in the trial. Many patients in either the treatment or control group who have a spontaneous remission of disease during the trial can make the new treatment look either too good or not bad at all.

Even if patients could be matched adequately in the two groups the further problem remains of assessing the effects of treatment which can make real comparison possible. Various scales have been devised to measure the amount of disability of a patient with MS. One is the Disability Status Scale (DSS) devised by Kurtzke. This scale assesses the amount of disease in various parts of the CNS and its effects on the body. Another, also devised by Kurtzke, is the Incapacity Scale which is more relevant to the impact of MS on the patient's daily life and activities. But it is still difficult to assess short-term improvement against long-term improvement with longer remissions and fewer and less frequent relapses, and to assess the well-being of the patient, which is impossible to measure in an objective way. In RCTs for other diseases the long-term effects can be measured by the length of life but this is not relevant in a chronic and variable disease such as MS. In MS there may be no measurable improvement during a trial of some therapy but, if the patient feels better, that alone may justify its use provided there are no serious side-effects. MS in many ways is a very 'individual' disease.

Corticotrophin and corticosteroids

There is no evidence that the long-term use of these drugs prevents relapses or alters the eventual outlook in MS, but they do speed up recovery from a relapse and improve the recovery rate. This is no longer a question of belief or disbelief because there is evidence of the shrinkage of observable lesions in the CNS using the CT scanner. There is no evidence that the use of steroids in an acute relapse will influence the extent of recovery. The CT scanner shows an arrest in the amount of oedema round a lesion and therefore steroids seem to be having an anti-inflammatory effect. An immunosuppressive effect is shown by the lowering of the amounts of protein and immunoglobulins in the CSF.

In practice, adrenocorticotrophic hormone (ACTH), which is a normal secretion from the pituitary gland, is given intramuscularly for the short term during a relapse. A typical course is twice daily injections for two to four weeks. There is no evidence that it is useful in long-term use and it can cause all the side-effects of steroid therapy including water retention, potassium loss, rounding of the face ('moonface') and diabetes. Corticosteroids, such as prednisone and prednisolone, can be given by mouth, intramuscularly or intravenously but are not the drugs of choice in an acute relapse. There is still no conclusive evidence that taken long-term these drugs can prevent relapses and maintain improvement. They may also inhibit the production of 'normal' corticosteroids by the body which does not occur with ACTH.

Neurologists may still have other views about the use of ACTH in acute relapses in spite of the objective evidence of their benefit from the CT scanner; and there are still some who do not believe in their use. Some will use 'depot' (long-acting) injections of ACTH which can be given less frequently and act for longer. Some people find that ACTH gives them a sense of well-being; others find that they get a 'high' which is not pleasant and can make sleep difficult. ACTH is accepted as useful and important when vision is affected and there is evidence of optic neuritis during an incident of MS or a relapse.

Immunosuppression

It is now widely known that immunosuppressants are used after transplant surgery to stop the body 'rejecting' or acting to kill off the transplanted organ. The possibility of MS having an immune type of cause has already been discussed. Theoretically, therefore, if a drug can be given that damps down this immune reaction of the body, which for the moment is acting against its own cells as it would do normally against foreign or invading cells, the rate of the destruction of the myelin sheaths could be slowed down and arrested before too much damage is done. The long-term effects of immunosuppression can be the development of certain cancers. Therefore, the benefits of such treatment must be good in order to outweigh the possible disadvantages.

One such drug is azathioprine (Imuran) which may be used in patients with frequent exacerbations or those suffering from a severe and progressive form of MS. The drug may be given continuously over a year or eighteen months and steroids added if relapses occur. Side-effects are less common with this drug than with cyclophosphamide which is more likely to cause cancer. The effects of this treatment can be shown by the CSF becoming more normal.

Plasmapheresis is replacement of the body plasma and hopefully of the substances which are involved in the auto-immune response. Although the concentration of immunoglobulins in the CSF may be lowered, the clinical results in MS during trials have been disappointing. Results during a trial in Australia of plasmapheresis and azathioprine were no better than with azathioprine alone.

Hyperbaric oxygen

Hyperbaric oxygen (HBO) was originally used in treating 'the bends' in deep-sea divers. The bends can occur in deep-sea divers who surface too quickly, and damage can be caused in the CNS similar to that found in MS. Divers have been treated by HBO since the 1930s for this disease. It was suggested that patients with MS should be treated in the same way and initial trials were encouraging. Patients are put in either a single chamber or in a larger multi-chamber designed to treat several patients at the same time. The door is sealed and the pressure in the chamber is raised by the introduction of air under pressure in the multi-chamber or oxygen under pressure in the single-patient chamber. In the multi-chamber patients breathe pure oxygen through a face mask for a period between twenty minutes and an hour. In the single chamber 100 per cent oxygen is already present so that the patient is already surrounded by as well as breathing it. The pressure is usually at least double normal atmospheric pressure.

There was great enthusiasm for this treatment and Action for Research into Multiple Sclerosis (ARMS) was instrumental in arranging for special HBO chambers to be available in many parts of the UK. However, a number of research papers in the *Lancet*, the *British Medical Journal*, the *New England Journal of Medicine* and the *Australian Medical Journal* have been published since 1983 showing that there is no evidence for improvement in MS by the use of HBO, but it is still used as a treatment because patients say that they feel better and feel that their MS has been improved, although this has not been demonstrated using conventional and scientifically acceptable ways of assessing improvement. ARMS has done some research on subjective as well as objective improvement; after all it is what the patient feels like that is of greatest interest to the patient! All the patients had full general physical and neurological assessments before the trial, and during the trial neither the doctors nor patients knew who was having oxygen and who air. The patients filled in two questionnaires. One was the Nottingham Health Profile in two parts, the first covering the common effects of ill health such as pain and social isolation, the second assessing the effects of ill health on specified activities. The General Health questionnaire asks for answers to questions about mental functioning and emotional well-being. Therefore the research included what the patients felt as well as what an external observer could measure. Though there were some improvements in patients with both the relapsing/remitting and chronic/progressive types of MS they were not great and were not maintained, but there were more improvements in the patients' assessments of themselves including energy and social well-being.

The *British Medical Journal* published a paper in February 1986

47

called 'Hyperbaric oxygen in multiple sclerosis: a double blind trial', and the abstract was as follows: eighty-four patients with MS were treated in monoplace chambers with either oxygen at two atmospheric pressures or placebo (air). Comprehensive double-blind assessment was carried out before, immediately after, and one month after treatment. There was no clinically important or significant benefit in any of the four major criteria of outcome – namely the patient's subjective opinion, the examiner's opinion, the score on the Kurtzke disability-status scale, or the time taken to walk fifty metres. Of forty other clinical variables assessed, two (the sensory scale and timed writing with the left hand) showed a significant improvement without any subjective clinical correlate or change in any of seven other tests of left-hand function. No group of symptoms was perceived by the patients as having improved more after treatment with hyperbaric oxygen than placebo.

It is concluded that there is no basis for recommending HBO in the treatment of MS.

It is difficult in any trial to eliminate the good and therapeutic effects of regular treatment and professional interest, or of regular outings and meeting with a group of people with the same interest in MS. One friend I know who had and still has HBO treatment says that she knows all about the scientific trials and that HBO has been shown of no value, but she adds that her outing to the HBO centre is the only time in her week when she meets people who understand the problems of MS, she is actually looked after and is given a cup of tea. Perhaps this description says a lot about the needs of MS people which HBO treatment is providing as a good side-effect. I think this could be called patient-orientated therapy and perhaps it is an example of the benefits which might arise by looking at the needs of the patients and how these needs could be supplied rather than at the pathology of MS and how it can be prevented or reversed, looked at from a scientifically orientated research angle.

Chapter 5 Diet

A whole book could be written about the various diets that have been advised for the management of MS. Alternatively the whole question of diet and MS could be written off by saying that no, definitely NO diet, has been proved to be of value in MS. So where does the truth lie and what are you going to do about your diet? All I can try to do here is sum up the present state of reliable knowledge on the subject of diet and refer you to books which may be of interest if you want to think further about the diet which will suit you best. I think that the last sentence sums up the right attitude to diet which you should think about and then cultivate. I shall add some of my own thoughts about diet and the need for self-care.

Perhaps it would be opportune to stress here that it is *your* body that has MS and it is important that you should feel as physically well as you possibly can and be able to cope as well as possible with the muscle weakness and fatigue which are such central parts of this teasing disease. Nobody knows the answer to the best diet because none has been proved to be of particular value. So it is important that you examine the evidence for the benefits of the one or the other and, provided that a diet is nutritionally sound and will not do you any harm, you are at liberty to experiment, preferably keep some sort of record, perhaps a food diary, and find out for yourself what sort of diet suits you best. Because MS can be such an unpleasant disease it is natural that patients should believe that a general practitioner or neurologist will know what is best for them, but I have doubts about this. A doctor who reads all the research papers about MS will know the current state of knowledge but beyond that he will not automatically know the best diet for you. Most doctors, apart from neurologists with a special interest in MS, will not have time to read all the research that is being done on MS, and it is quite possible that you will be better informed than your general practitioner, and as there is no proof that any diet is the best diet, it is up to you to discover which diet makes you feel fittest. It is what you feel in your own body and mind that is the most important thing and it is very easy for doctors and patients to forget that. I believe that a little of what you fancy really does do you good! Provided that you are totally honest about your own physical and mental feelings.

When I was thinking about diet before starting this book I read many different types of diet theories, including those for cancer, arthritis and heart disease. I was quite surprised to find the number of things that they had in common. Yes, there are differences but on the whole there are many more things in common than things different. I began to feel that we are really talking about a diet for good health as we understand it at the end of the twentieth century. MS is one of the 'degenerative diseases' which have appeared in Western civilization during the past two hundred years or so and is almost certainly tied up with changes in our ways of living and eating since the Industrial Revolution. Before I describe the diets that have been recommended for MS I shall look at some of the changes in diet that have occurred during the past two centuries.

One of the biggest changes has been in the consumption of sugar. Sugar was not generally available in the UK until the eighteenth century when it was imported from the British West Indies. Before that it had come from the Mediterranean ports and was a luxury item. During the eighteenth century the per capita consumption of sugar rose seven-and-a-half times, and consumption of tea and coffee increased. The importing of sugar was at that time an integral part of the slave trade. We eat now the same amount of sugar in two weeks as we ate in a year two hundred years ago, and we eat five times as much sugar now as we ate a hundred years ago. With increasing material prosperity the amount of fat and protein in the diet increases, but the carbohydrate content falls – apart from sugar – and that increases markedly. It is easy to say that you do not eat much sugar, meaning that you do not add sugar to tea or coffee, but you will be eating a lot of sugar, not only in puddings, ice-cream, confectionery, cake and biscuits but in all the hidden ways. If you look at the contents of tinned and frozen foods, including vegetables and savouries, you will see how many of them contain sugar. In recent years there has been a move away from this and you will find many tins of fruit or cereals labelled 'with no added sugar'. It is a step in the right direction but we are a sweet-eating nation – the Scots most particularly.

These are only personal observations and I do not expect to prove anything or be taken seriously because I am only writing about one patient in this instance, and that is myself. But I do know that sugar and any sugar-containing food does me no good. I enjoy eating sweet food but tend to eat more than I want once I have started – and tend to feel hungry soon afterwards and want more to eat. If I eat a lot of sweet food not only do I get indigestion but some hours later I have a fast heart rate, feel a bit sweaty and generally anxious. I am not a diabetic and I do not regularly sit and count my heart rate! It is only after many years of these feelings that the connection with sugar has dawned on me and avoiding sugar prevents my having the symptoms; I also feel better and more energetic and sleep better. Of course, physiologically, eating sugar causes a rapid rise in insulin and I wonder if this is what for me appears to produce a sort of mild and brief anxiety state. Perhaps the swing between high and low levels of blood sugar and insulin produce recurrent internal stresses in the body. I am no physiologist but I do know how I feel! Perhaps some of the readers of this book will be interested to try avoiding sugar and let me know their observations. A great deal of work has been done on fat in the diet and it would be interesting to look at the consumption of sugar in the areas where MS has a high incidence.

Obesity is never good, and particularly in a disease which has muscle weakness as an essential part. Obesity also encourages the development of bronchitis, heart disease, arthritis and diabetes, so the message is that obesity and physical fitness are incompatible. If you are not able to move around, weight gain is likely to be a problem because you will actually need much less food. If you are feeling low because you are getting less mobile, you may crave food for comfort and a vicious circle can so easily be created. Perhaps we should look at the diets for obesity first because everybody agrees that obesity is not healthy, particularly if you have MS.

Which diet for obesity?

Crash diets are not advisable. The advertising for any crash diet may be very alluring but it is not the answer to a chronic weight problem. You may lose weight immediately but it will go on again and it is possible that the next lot of fat that you add to your body may be even more difficult to lose than the last lot; and that is a depressing thought. I have certainly found it to be so. Crash diets do not help you to eat more sensibly in the longer term. I find that the Scarsdale diet, which has been around for many years, is a suitable one for losing weight and re-educating myself to eat more sensibly. It recommends the cutting of fat in the diet and you can change the balance between saturated and unsaturated fats if you wish. It is worth buying the book on the Scarsdale diet (*The Complete Scarsdale Medical Diet* by Herman Tarnower and Samm Sinclair Baker) if you are going to try it. You are instructed to keep strictly to the diet for fourteen days only and then go on to a maintenance diet. I enjoy the diet, feel well on it and I lose weight – if I stick to it. But you may not find it as helpful, or be prepared to give up some of the banned foods such as butter and margarine. If this is so you must try and find the right diet for yourself. You may be someone who needs a lot of support in order to reduce your weight, so you may find it helpful to join a group for weight reduction. Or perhaps you could organize a local group of people with MS or other conditions which reduce mobility and make a weight problem more difficult to solve. Obesity is not a problem which somebody else can solve for you, in spite of yourself as it were. A doctor can give you a diet sheet but cannot see that you stick to it and that you do not eat a lot of additional food.

There is a rather nice book claiming to help you beat temptations and get slim. *The Dieter's Guide to Success* is written by Audrey Eyton and Dr Henry Jordan and I have found a lot of help in its pages. There is a gem on the subject of leftovers.

> While we are struggling to shed weight, visitors coming to our home often provide us with an excellent excuse to cook the foods we are tending to avoid because we find them so tempting. Here's an excellent, personally acceptable reason to bake that cake or make those biscuits! Here's a great temptation to eat much more

of them than we ever estimated. The common tendency in catering for visitors is to overestimate rather than underestimate the quantity of food that will be required. No one wants to risk not having sufficient food to offer. What this usually leaves us with after the visit is leftovers of a particularly tempting nature. What we usually do is consume them ourselves eating much more superfluous food after the visitors have left than while we were eating with them.

The suggested solutions are offering the leftovers to the visitors or freezing them.

I think that it is this sort of approach to problem solving with regard to food that will help you do something about shedding surplus weight. The idea of being a helpless victim of your own fat and that it is the responsibility of your doctor to get rid of it for you is palpably nonsense; but it is so easy to fail to recognize the problems that are ours and for which we must be responsible if they are to be solved. If you do not own up to the problem it is going to be difficult to get help and that is true for many health problems.

A low-fat diet will help you to reduce weight and this diet may also be your choice long-term for managing your life with MS. When fat is metabolized in the body it produces twice as many calories as either protein or carbohydrate from the same weight of food. A reduction in fat can therefore produce a large drop in calories. A gluten-free diet can also be weight-reducing but this will happen largely because it is not an appetizing diet. If you do choose a gluten-free diet you may find weight loss a welcome side-effect.

Unlike me you may thrive on a calorie-controlled diet with weighing of every item, or you may prefer to fast one day a week. The choice is enormous but it is up to you to find the way that is right for you. There is no proof of a best way or one which works for everybody. Listen to your own body. If necessary learn more about dietary requirements, discuss the facts with a person who is knowledgeable about diet and then make your own decisions and go on listening to your own body.

How fast should you lose weight? It is a mistake to lose it too fast. A steady weight loss of about one-and-a-half to two pounds a week (approximately 0.5–1.0kg) is ideal. You will probably have to keep an eye on your weight indefinitely but you may well find that once you have shed all the surplus fat you can relax a bit.

For sticking to a diet I find the Alcoholics Anonymous approach of 'just for today' helpful; and my own inner mutterings of 'only once won't make any difference' totally unhelpful. If you think about giving up alcohol, or limiting your food, for life it seems an impossible task; but 'just for today' is more acceptable and manageable.

The low-fat diet

A low-fat or non-animal-fat diet was first described by the US physician Dr R. L. Swank and his first work on the diet was done at McGill University, Montreal, in 1948. His book has been republished and is interesting to read. Many neurologists and other doctors give him credit for this earliest work on what is still a medically acceptable diet, but he is criticized for publishing the results and basing a theory on relatively few treated patients. He observed that in areas of the world where the total intake of fat in the diet is less than 24g a day the incidence of MS is low and in areas where the daily fat is high and possibly even 150g a day the incidence of MS is higher. He made the distinction between hard fats, which are set at room temperature, and soft fats or oils, which are runny at room temperature. In his first trial with MS patients the limits on daily intake were 15g for hard fat and 20g for oil. He decided that oils did no harm and subsequently raised the upper daily intake of oil to 50g.

Oils and fats can be described more scientifically as saturated fats and unsaturated fats, the latter being divided into mono-unsaturated and polyunsaturated fats. The difference is in the formula, which is complicated: in the mono-unsaturated fats there is one carbon atom in the molecule, held together by a double bond instead of a single bond, while in the polyunsaturated fats there are two or more carbon atoms linked in this way, and in the saturated fats there are no double bonds. The double bond increases the activity in the body. The saturated fats are the animal fats and other fats which are solid at room temperature such as the more conventional types of margarine. It is the polyunsaturated fats that appear to be most desirable in people with MS. A number of theories have been put forward and continue to be put forward to account for this phenomenon, but in general it seems that a higher concentration of polyunsaturated fat in the blood protects the nerve sheaths from whatever it is that initiates their demyelination in MS.

In proteins there are essential amino acids and they are the ones that the body is unable to synthesize and which need to be present in the diet. In a similar way in fats there are essential fatty acids (EFAs) and these are linoleic, linolenic and arachidonic acids. These are of particular importance in the nervous system and for the repair of damaged nerve tissue. There is evidence that some people with MS are not able to metabolize these fats correctly in the body and that there are lower than normal levels of them in the CNS. Foods rich in linoleic acid are sunflower seed oil, safflower seed oil, liver and kidneys. Foods rich in linolenic oil are fish, fish liver oils and green vegetables. In the normal body, gamma-linolenic acid is produced from linolenic acid, but in the person with MS this may not take place. The oil of the evening primrose plant is particularly rich in this oil and it has been recommended for patients with MS. Again it must be stressed that its benefit has not been proved scientifically, but it can do no harm and is worth trying. There is evidence that zinc may help the body use the EFAs in the diet and this can be bought as tablets. The oil is available in capsules, but it is fairly expensive and is not available on NHS prescription in the UK. To work most effectively the capsules should be taken with Vitamins C, B_6, E and a zinc supplement.

Much research continues to be done on the EFAs, their metabolism in the body and the part they play in MS. Both the MS Society and ARMS will keep you informed in their publications about the latest research work and its possible practical application for those with MS.

The following tables have been reproduced from my book *The Low-fat Gourmet* (Pelham, 1980; paperback, Sphere, 1980). The tables give some idea of the suitable foods to use if you are going to try the low-fat diet, but it is important to realize that you are not undertaking a regime that is going to cure MS. This is not a crash diet but one that you may choose to live with for many years. It is, therefore, important to make it as acceptable to your palate as possible and also make it fit in with family cooking and eating as much as possible.

Table Two: Amounts of fat and oil in commonly used foods

Food	Approximate portion containing 5g/1 teaspoon fat		Approximate portion containing 5g/1 teaspoon oil	
Fish	g	oz	g	oz
Cod	225	8	225	8
Crab	150	6	100	4
Haddock				
fresh	225	8	300	12
smoked	225	8	225	8
Halibut	100	4	50	2
Herring				
fresh	25	1	25	1
pickled	25	1		
smoked	50	2		
Lobster	225	8	225	8
Mackerel				
fresh	50	2	100	4
smoked	50	2		
Mussels	225	8	225	8
Salmon	50	2	150	6
Shrimps	225	8	225	8
Trout	225	8		
Tuna	25	1	50	2

Vegetables

Most vegetables contain minimal amounts of fat and oil and can be eaten in an unlimited quantity provided that fat is not used in their preparation. Chips are banned. The following are exceptions.

	g	oz	g	oz
Broad beans	225	8		
Soya beans	75	3	50	2

Fruit

Nearly all fruit may be eaten in unlimited quantities because it contains negligible amounts of fat and oil. The following are exceptions.

Food	Approximate portion containing 5g/l teaspoon fat		Approximate portion containing 5g/l teaspoon oil	
	g	oz	g	oz
Avocado pear	225	8	225	8
Olives	50	2		

Nuts

Almonds	10	½	50	2
Brazils	10	½	25	1
Chestnuts	500	16		
Cashews	10	½	225	8
Hazelnuts	10	½	25	1
Peanuts	25	1	50	2
Walnuts	50	2	10	½

Cereals

Bread				
pumpernickel	350	12		
white	225	8		
Flour				
buckwheat	225	8		
maize	225	8		
rye	350	12		
white	350	12		
wholemeal	225	8		
Oat flakes	225	8	225	8
Rice				
brown	350	12		
polished	500	16		
Semolina				
maize	350	12		
wheat	500	16		
Wheatgerm	50	2	225	8

Fats

Butter	*Avoid*			
Cheese				
Cheddar	25	1		
cream	25	1		

Food	Approximate portion containing 5g/1 teaspoon fat		Approximate portion containing 5g/1 teaspoon oil	
	g	oz		
Emmental	25	1		
Mozzarella	35	1½		
Parmesan	25	1		
skimmed cottage	225	8		
Eggs				
whole	1 egg		1 egg	
white	Unlimited			
yolk	25g	1oz		
Lard	Avoid			
Margarine				
ordinary	Avoid			
polyunsaturated fat (PUF)	25g	1oz	5g	¼oz
Milk				
whole	50ml	2oz		
dried skimmed	Unlimited			
Oil				
corn	Avoid			
olive	Avoid			
safflower			5g	1 teaspoon
sunflower-seed (SFS)			5g	1 teaspoon
Yoghurt				
commercial low-fat	225g	8oz		
home-made skimmed	Unlimited			

Meat	g	oz
Bacon, lean	25	1
Beef, lean	50	2
Chicken, without skin	100	4
Ham, lean	25	1
Hare	225	8
Heart, lean	75	3

Food	Approximate portion containing 5g/1 teaspoon fat		Approximate portion containing 5g/1 teaspoon oil
	g	oz	
Kidney	150	6	
Lamb, lean leg	75	3	
Liver	150	6	
Rabbit	150	6	
Turkey, without skin	100	6	
Venison	225	8	

If you do decide to try this diet it may be helpful to see a dietician, or join ARMS and get their excellent literature on the subject.

In general you should avoid the following completely: whole milk, butter, cream, margarine, cheese (except low-fat cottage cheese), chocolate, lard and anything containing any of these foods.

An average helping of lean meat may be taken once a day or less often; eggs, if eaten at all, should be limited to two a week. The white of egg can be eaten in moderation.

Low-fat cottage cheese and plenty of white fish or shellfish should be eaten to keep up your protein intake.

Food, where possible, should be grilled rather than fried.

Oil, when used for cooking or making mayonnaise or French dressing, should be sunflower seed oil. You will probably find that when it is used in cooking for the family nobody will notice any change of flavour. If oil is used for frying it should not be over-heated and never re-used. You can use margarine which is labelled as containing polyunsaturated fat either on your bread or in cooking.

If you are going to keep to a low-fat diet you should eat a maximum daily amount of 15g/½oz of fat and a minimum of 20g/¾oz of oil. Therefore it is more important to know the fat content of the food than the oil content provided that you are taking a required minimum of oil each day.

Yoghurt

I find that low-fat natural yoghurt is a great standby for puddings and for use instead of soured cream in the preparation of salads, vegetables and fish dishes. The best way of making it is in the airing cupboard. I usually start with a Greek yoghurt that I like but any 'live' yoghurt can be used. Bring a quart of skimmed milk to the boil and then allow it to simmer for about a minute. Remove from the heat and allow it to cool to blood temperature. Whisk two tablespoons of the 'starter' yoghurt on its own in a separate bowl and then into the cooled milk. Cover the bowl with clingfilm, wrap a towel round it and put it in the airing cupboard overnight. Any other reasonably warm place would do.

If you cut too much fat out of your diet you may start feeling tired and hungry and you may also be taking too low a number of calories. To counteract this you will probably have to increase the amount of protein and to some extent the amount of carbohydrate in your food. I find that it is helpful to use whole cereals and I bake my own bread. Beans and peas, soya beans, buckwheat, cracked wheat and freshly sprouted seeds are all ways of increasing my protein intake without increasing either the fat content or the expense of the diet. If you cut almost all animal fat out of your diet and you do not like margarine it is important to supplement your Vitamin A and D intake but I shall deal with this under vitamins.

The Essential Fatty Acid Diet

This is a modification of the Swank low-fat diet, based on research done in the UK by Dr Michael Crawford and is recommended by ARMS. Good accounts of the diet can be read in the ARMS literature and in Judy Graham's book, *Multiple Sclerosis*.

In the ARMS booklet *Diet Rich in Essential Fatty Acids* it gives the general rules of the diet:

1 Use polyunsaturated margarine and oils.

2 Eat at least three helpings of fish a week.

3 Eat ½lb liver a week.

4 Eat a large helping of dark green vegetables daily.

5 Eat some raw vegetables daily, as a salad with French dressing.

6 Eat some linseeds or Linusit Gold (a brand of split linseeds available from health food shops) daily.

7 Eat some fresh fruit daily.

8 Try to eat as much fresh food as possible in preference to processed food.

9 Choose lean cuts of meat, and trim all the fat away from the meat before cooking.

10 Try to avoid hard animal fats like butter, lard, suet, dripping, and fatty foods such as cream, hard cheese, etc.

11 Try to eat wholegrain cereals and wholemeal bread rather than refined cereals.

12 Try to cut down on sugar and foods containing sugar.

This seems to me to be a sensible diet which is in line with healthy living whether you have MS or not. A normal family diet could be based on it and I am happy about the censure on sugar; I have already written about sugar because I believe it could be not just undesirable in the diet but possibly harmful. In this booklet it describes sugar as bad because it provides calories without nutrition – what has sometimes been described as 'naked calories'. It does not, however, mention my own idea that the danger of sugar is in the fluctuating blood sugar level and the internal stresses which this may produce in the body.

ARMS can provide recipes based on this dietary advice. I think that it is important not to go round talking about your diet or expecting a hostess to cater for you, certainly not for one or two meals. It is easy to omit butter, milk and cream from most meals set before you without any problems for your hostess, or indeed anybody noticing. It does not matter if you do eat some food which you normally would not because you must remember that this diet is not a proven cure for MS. There are variations on this diet including one which allows dairy products providing they are fresh. I think it is up to you to experiment and find the diet on which you feel fittest and then stick to that one.

The gluten-free diet

A gluten-free diet is used primarily for children or adults who have coeliac disease; for them such a diet is essential for the rest of their lives. Gluten is the harmful part of the protein in wheat, rye and barley and therefore all these cereals must be avoided. A very small amount of gluten will be harmful. Bread and any other foods must be made with gluten-free flour and a careful watch kept on all ready-prepared foods used, such as tinned foods, sauces, ketchups and gravies. The person with coeliac disease knows that eating gluten is incompatible with good or even reasonably good health, and this in itself is usually sufficient incentive to remain on the diet. The patient with MS does not have the same certainty but if he feels that such a diet might help him, few doctors would try to dissuade him. One idea which supported a possibility of the gluten theory was the high flour and, therefore, gluten intake in the north of Scotland and the Orkney Islands where MS has its highest reported incidence in the world. Another was the belief that the same changes were found in the small intestine of people with MS as in those of patients with coeliac disease, but this has now been disapproved.

Roger MacDougall is a writer who developed MS and became severely disabled. He disappeared from the writing world and was later tracked down by a curious journalist. He had put himself on a gluten-free diet and also eliminated coffee and alcohol from his diet. He seemed to have made a remarkable recovery and was able to move about freely again and to lead a full and normal life. Neurologists examined him and found signs still of MS but that he was now well and mobile.

Following the first publication of this story there were, quite naturally, nationwide inquiries at neurological departments about this new 'cure' for MS. The neurologists knew nothing about it but many patients went on the diet because at least it could do them no harm. A neurologist undertook a trial of the gluten-free diet with forty-two patients. Five dropped out of the trial because they found the food unpalatable: of the remainder who stayed on it for the length of the trial there was no evidence that their symptoms improved or that they were less likely to have a relapse. Following this trial few neurologists would recommend a gluten-free diet but there are still patients who wish to try it and some seem to benefit.

The diet as recommended now also advises a reduction in the amounts of refined sugar and saturated fats and the addition of a mineral and vitamin supplement in addition to the restrictions on gluten. Roger MacDougall remained well and active, has written a book, *My Fight Against Multiple Sclerosis* and also markets his own blend of vitamin and mineral supplement.

Other diets

There have been other descriptions of miraculous results with diet and some of these include ideas about allergy to food. Descriptions of food allergies and testing for them can be read in the books *Not All in the Mind* and *Chemical Victims* by Richard Mackarness. He describes his work as clinical ecology and it is not directly referable to MS; but for any readers who are interested in the idea of food allergy these books provide interesting reading.

Rita Greer's husband Alan was severely crippled with MS and Rita found that he was better without meat in his diet. By a process of trial and error she worked out the foods that were bad and the ones that were good for him. During this time many stresses were removed from his life. He made a remarkable recovery and was able to abandon his wheelchair and walking aids. Of course, the medical profession does not find it easy to accept such cures based on the experience of one person and which cannot usually be repeated under more scientific conditions. But I have no doubt that he did make a remarkable recovery and Rita Greer's *Extraordinary Kitchen Notebook* makes interesting reading. Alan remained on a vegan diet for about four years and this would not suit some people. I believe that the common factor in the accounts of such surprising 'cures' is that the patient finds a diet and usually a lifestyle which is right for him. Such changes may be applicable to other people, particularly such items as a 'healthier' diet and relief from stresses, but I believe that such changes are 'bespoke' and cannot be taken 'off the peg' and used by another person. They should be studied and thought about. If there are factors which do fit you then it might be worth making the same or similar changes. But each person is unique and therefore what is right for one person may not be right for you. Self-knowledge and understanding are most important and a slavish adherence to some diet or regime that was right for somebody else is not necessarily going to be as beneficial for you.

Is a diet worth while?

There is no easy answer to this question. Some neurologists recommend a diet; others may say that they do not believe it helps and therefore do not suggest one. I think the answer is to understand some of the modern ideas about diet which are recommended both to avoid heart attacks and 'treat' MS. A reduction in weight is always advisable – but not to the point of becoming underweight. Sugar can be almost eliminated from a diet and its disappearance will do nothing but good. A lowering in the total amount of fat in the diet with particular emphasis on the reduction of saturated fat will also be beneficial for your general physical health. I do not believe that a slavish adherence to any particular diet for MS is necessarily good.

What about vitamin and mineral supplements?

Many claims have been made for various vitamins and their benefits. At one time Vitamin B_{12} was used as injections in the treatment of MS but again there is no scientific evidence that it helps. It is used in the treatment of pernicious anaemia. Some people with MS do still have injections and feel that they benefit.

Once again it is important to stress that there is no scientific proof that any particular blend of vitamins and minerals will 'cure' MS or even be best in its management. You can either take a multivitamin and mineral daily supplement or concentrate on some of the vitamins and minerals. Vitamins C, B compound and E have all had special claims made for their value. Your intake of Vitamins A and D may be reduced if you are cutting out butter, and all other dairy products and margarine. It is important that you do not take too much Vitamin A and it will be unwise to take a supplement of cod liver oil if you are taking some vitamins in your diet and a multivitamin tablet.

I would suggest as a general guide: take one multivitamin and mineral tablet daily and supplement this with a tablet of zinc, or the recommended amount as given on the bottle. I find that a large dose of Vitamin C daily, that is 2g, does seem to help me avoid colds, and there is no doubt that frequent virus infections, such as colds, can cause an exacerbation of MS symptoms.

This is a brief summary of a reasonable daily vitamin and mineral supplement. You can, if you wish, add sunflower seed oil either as liquid or in capsules. I suggest that you read some of the literature on the subject of vitamin and mineral supplements if you feel that this would be of interest to you; and then make your own decision on what you will take. Once again I stress that there is no known daily amount of dietary supplements that will cure MS. It is important for you to think about getting as physically fit as possible so that you can concentrate on leading your own life creatively.

Chapter 6   *Physiotherapy and Physical Fitness*

Physiotherapy and regular exercise need to be thought about and used together towards achieving general physical fitness. They could become enjoyable parts of your daily life. You may say that you have never been an athletic person and now that you have MS it is hardly the right time to start. But doing some work towards getting a fitter body can be fun and you will find it easier to like your body again when it feels an abler servant for what you want to do. Physiotherapy and exercise must not be looked on as school subjects that are not quite connected with real life. They are two more tools that you can use in achieving better health.

There is no one right or best way to use physiotherapy in the management of MS and the value of organized physiotherapy on a regular basis is doubtful. For most patients and most physiotherapists, unless the patient is in hospital, a short regular daily session is impossible. Irregular lengthy sessions may be too tiring at the time and not be repeated sufficiently often at home afterwards. One solution seems to be that exercises should be taught by a physiotherapist as required, or possibly as recommended by the doctor after discussion with the patient, and these should then be worked on quietly at home on a regular basis. Occasional visits should be made to the physiotherapist for supervision or for working out new exercises. If money, or possibly lack of money, is not too pressing a problem it may be a good idea to see a physiotherapist privately on an irregular basis so that you can see her when you want to, rather than when she can manage to fit you in, which can happen in a busy hospital out-patient department.

My first exercises were worked out with the help of my athlete son and were geared to strenthening all my limbs. I found that exercises to stretch the backs of my legs were very difficult at first but could be managed much more easily in a warm bath. I have often needed to do exercises to strengthen my left arm and leg. At times I have had to work hard to stop my left wrist remaining flexed forward. I tend not to use my left hand a lot because it is clumsy and so it can remain for long periods bent forward. I need to remember to exercise it when I am sitting doing nothing much; and that is not a regular occurrence! These are only my own personal examples and will probably have nothing to do with your problems at the moment. I write about them only to give you the idea of using any help that is available to you in such a way as to get the maximum benefit from it. I think the most sensible way is to exercise regularly but to concentrate on the parts of your body that seem to be in particular need at any one time.

I find the ARMS approach to physiotherapy interesting. The patient is first asked what he wants to be able to achieve and his physiotherapy is then geared towards this achievement. In the course of MS, muscles are weakened because their nerve supply is affected and in rehabilitation there will be an element of making the best use of muscle power that remains as well as re-education so that you can teach your muscles a new way of achieving the same goal. For instance if you want to get from lying to standing you can either attempt to strengthen existing muscles so that you can achieve the whole operation while remaining with your back down; or you can learn a new way of getting from prone to upright by first turning on to your front and then getting on to your feet. That is a very simple example and probably one that many people with MS have learnt by instinct because it is embarrassing not to be able to get to a standing position without help. ARMS calls this maintaining independence in the activities of daily living (ADLs). This is a special sort of physiotherapy which is geared individually and it is the patient who decides the aims and their priorities. I believe it is this element of choice and the patient-centred approach which can make this system effective in maintaining mobility and independence.

The ARMS principles of physiotherapy for MS patients include the following guide-lines:

1 Encourage development of strategies of movement.

2 Encourage learning of motor skills.

3 Improve the quality of patterns of movement.

4 Minimize abnormalities of muscle tone.

5 Emphasize the functional application of therapy.

6 Support the patient to maintain motivation and co-operation and to reinforce therapy.

7 Implement preventive therapy.

8 Educate patients re the above, for coping with everyday life.

I hope that ARMS will not become too 'scientific' in their descriptions of what they are trying to do and be content to keep all their treatment individually oriented and go at the pace that the patient dictates. One of the problems of the scientific approach and presentation is that it can disguise the importance of the 'à la carte' approach which stresses the uniqueness of each person with MS. Science wants statistics about MS patients, but the people who have MS want ways of coping with their individual problems.

What sort of exercise?

You need to do the sort of exercise which makes you feel good and finding out what that is may mean some trial and error. It must not be exercise of the sort and in the amount that leaves you exhausted and demoralized. So it will depend to a certain extent on the sort of exercise to which you were accustomed before you developed MS. It will probably be difficult to go on with any sport that requires speed in running or a good sense of balance. But there are plenty of physical activities which require neither. It is important that you find one which you enjoy, can do regularly and which makes you feel better. Walking or cycling are both good forms of exercise. Swimming can be excellent and can be useful for increasing the mobility of stiff arms and legs. Whatever you choose to do it is important that you do it because you want to do it and you feel some benefit from it. It must not become just one more chore to get through in a dull life. Try to find something that really does make you feel more mentally and physically alive and which gives you pleasure.

There is a small book published by Penguin called *Physical Fitness* which gives useful schemes of exercises and it gives plans which can be done in eleven minutes daily for men and twelve minutes daily for women. These are based on exercises devised by the Royal Canadian Air Force and all the exercises are geared to your age and present state of fitness. These exercises, I agree, can be more a question of discipline than enjoyment; but when I do them regularly, which is not often, they make me feel so much better that the reward is great after a few days of work.

A neurologist who laid much stress on exercise and a particular sort of exercise was W. Ritchie Russell, formerly a Professor of Clinical Neurology at Oxford. In 1976 he published a book called *Multiple Sclerosis – Control of the Disease*, which is no longer given any publicity. He believed that the course of MS can be influenced by the amount of blood supplied to the brain and improving what he called 'the blood brain barrier'. Push-ups, he felt, are the most effective form of exercise because they improve the circulation, particularly in the upper part of the body, neck and brain, and worked out a regime for each patient which he firmly believed could have not only a marked influence on the current state of MS but also on the long-term relapses. This regime needed to be followed for an indefinite period of time. Each patient would be assessed and given a timetable with the prescribed number of push-ups to be done at a stated number of times a day and a precise amount of rest to be taken after each lot of exercise.

If you can get hold of a copy of this book, it makes interesting reading. I think the idea of a twice-daily period of exercise until sweating slightly, followed by a period of rest, is probably a very good one; there may also be some benefit in increasing the blood circulation in the head and neck areas. I do not find, however, that I get the most benefit from one particular exercise repeated for an indefinite period but rather from different exercises at different times according to the needs of the moment. This sort of programme ties in with the current ideas about the need for anaerobic exercise to achieve physical fitness; so if you are the sort of person who can be committed to two regular spells of push-ups a day, this scheme might be beneficial.

A housewife will say that she does not need any additional exercise because she can always find some sort of activity around the house, but housework is not necessarily the best exercise and is not likely to cover all the body movements that need to be done. It may be more fun to have two brisk walks a day or go swimming on a regular basis.

What about yoga?

Yoga may be a most important sort of activity for somebody with MS and I am sorry that, so far, I have not tried it. I believe it is important because it stresses the interlinking of body, mind and spirit and also it gives more emphasis to the things we are able to do rather than allowing us to brood on the things which we can no longer do. MS is a type of bereavement, and it is all too easy to shut oneself up with one's own sadness and build barriers against friends and the feelings which could be healing. Yoga is a way of being put back in touch with one's own body and can help rekindle the 'life-force' which can make us feel really alive again. The phrase 'the breath of life' is a significant one and by helping with breathing and control of the diaphragm, I believe that yoga can be a powerful force for good. In 1978 the MS Society was involved in setting up the Yoga for Health Foundation in Bedfordshire. Many people with MS have stayed there and found it most helpful. Perhaps part of the importance is that yoga is not a competitive activity and aims at relaxation and energy control. For those who are not able to get to classes or go to a course at the Yoga for Health Foundation, there is a tape, *Yoga and Multiple Sclerosis* or a book, *Yoga for the Disabled* available from the Foundation and the address is in the Appendix.

Chapter 7 MS Fatigue and its Management

What is so special about MS fatigue?

Everyone gets tired sometimes so what is different about getting tired if you have MS? I think that MS fatigue is a special sort of tiredness and it is partly due to the damage that has been done in the CNS. A frightening exacerbation of MS symptoms can occur during a time of fatigue; but there is not necessarily a change in the physical signs on examination. This disparity between what the patient feels and what the doctor finds is one of the mysterious things in MS; and it does not mean that the patient is 'putting it on'. However, sometimes severe fatigue can precipitate a relapse with worsening of both symptoms and signs. Fatigue does seem to be both a cause and a result of MS and learning to live with it is important.

Learning to live at a reasonable speed, with sufficient and regular rest and avoiding undue fatigue is an art. I am sure that it can be acquired quite easily by some people, but I am not among them and perhaps all those with MS have this difficulty. If I feel well I forget all about MS as far as possible and spend several days doing very much more than is reasonable, or drive some ridiculous distance in a car. Recently the problem has been too many hours in front of my word processor with my eyes glued to a VDU and my back in an awkward position. Technology changes fast but wisdom grows so slowly! By the time fatigue has caught up with me I am unable to sleep properly because of spasms in my leg muscles and aching back muscles and it can then take several weeks, when I am forced to limit my activity, before I am functioning well again. It is very stupid because more of one's life can be used profitably if one learns to ration one's activity.

Avoiding fatigue is not only important for you but also for your family, friends and workmates. Fatigue not only makes you feel bad but it spreads around you and affects other people with whom you come in contact; and it is your responsibility to learn how much you can manage without getting overtired. This could need a lot of thought about your priorities.

Changing some habits

You will need to look at the things in your life that tend to bring on severe fatigue. It may be travelling in a car or on the train, hot baths, arguments at home especially about money, frustrations at work or cooking in a hot kitchen. It is impossible to give all the possible causes because MS is a variable disease and each person with it is unique. It is up to you to look at your own body, mind and lifestyle. For me, late nights and too much coffee are frequently precipitants of trouble. A few long nights, some regular gentle exercise and more thought about my body are the restorers; but again there are no hard and fast 'rules' about this and you must learn to be aware of and 'listen' to your own body. It does seem important in MS to have regular periods of rest and exercise.

What sort of rest?

At times of acute fatigue after making a long journey or just being generally overactive I find that for me a few inactive days can bring about a remarkable improvement. A day or two in bed may be necessary. Dr Swank recommended that all patients with MS should take a regular rest in the middle of the day and that it should be increased to twice a day during bad patches. To manage this a housewife with young children needs to become as competent in administering her time and energy as a company director in running his firm. It helps if you are not too obsessional about housework and are capable of leaving the washing-up if you need a break.

During an acute relapse you may be advised to have a spell of complete rest. If you are unable to do this at home, it may be suggested that you go into hospital for a while. A mother with young children may find it impossible to make arrangements so that she can get sufficient rest at home, but most women find that with adequate help, home is the best place to be when very tired. I have found that a hospital bed is one of the least restful places to be, even in a single room. There seems to be some sort of noise going on around the clock. Sleep can be disturbed by the devilish device of a glass panel over a door and a bright light left on outside. I have found that even if I dropped off during the day somebody would arrive and want a blood sample. Perhaps the most peaceful hospitals and nursing homes are those run by religious orders. Sadly there are not many of these.

What are you going to do while you rest?

The most important thing is to choose the right place where you can relax completely. Try to choose a warm corner – perhaps with a view. When I wrote my last book about MS I rested in a room with a magnificent view over the Moray Firth in the north of Scotland. Now I live in a small mid-terrace house in a city centre. I no longer have the advantage of a glorious view outside so I must make my own view inside: a particular painting gives me a great sense of peace and sometimes I light a candle and look at the stillness of the flame. Now a relax-style chair is a great help to me, but you may prefer to lie on cushions on the floor or on your bed. There are plenty of options and you must find the one that helps you most. Perhaps television or quiet music will help; or you may be able to sleep and that can be very good. One of my current schemes for getting more physical rest is to take a thermos of coffee to bed with me and drink it next morning while I spend an extra hour or two in bed writing.

At any time during the day when you sit down try to put your feet up and relax completely even if it is only for a matter of minutes. There is an art in doing the maximum amount of work with the least expenditure of energy. You must not waste energy by standing around talking or just pottering around unless pottering is exactly what you are wanting to do at a given moment. I keep a stool by the telephone so that I need not waste effort standing and during a long telephone call I slip quietly on to the floor and lie flat on my back and relax.

Organizing a routine

It helps to make some sort of routine for yourself if you know you are going to spend a while at home either when you are first diagnosed or later during a relapse. You do not have to stick to the routine rigidly but having some sort of plan for your day may help you feel less anxious. Decide when your mealtimes will be and think about what you are going to eat. Whether you actually feel hungry or not, prepare and eat your food at approximately the time you had arranged. Try not to drink too many cups of tea and coffee; they may make you feel more tense and possibly interfere with sleep. You could try decaffeinated coffee or herb tea. Make sure you have a rest time. But do not necessarily do what I have suggested here; it is much more important that you begin to regain control over your own time, energy, mind and body. By assuming responsibility for yourself in this way I believe there is a better chance of remaining healthy and reasonably active for a longer time.

I have found it helpful to have some time each day planned for activities such as writing letters, listening to the radio or music and watching television. The *Radio Times* and *TV Times* can become interesting reading when you are planning the things that you really want to hear and see and actually have time to do both. Doing and thinking about the things that give you real pleasure matters at this juncture in your life. You must change course if you are going to become healthier, and this is the interval when you can begin to think positively about your own future. The medical 'take-over' of your health, your body and your future should be only temporary and any medical intervention should be helpful and acceptable to you. But you must remember that it is your body and your life and you do have the right to accept what is helpful and reject what is not helpful.

Reading books can be recreational particularly if you have been doing a full-time job and have not had the mental energy to read, or have been bringing up a family and may have got out of the habit of reading. You might start reading book reviews and pick out one or two that you think would interest you and get them from the library, or you can ask the librarian to recommend a book. It might be a good idea to join one of the well-run book clubs and have the pleasure of choosing a number of books each year that you can afford to buy and have time to read. As you discover the feeling of the books that you really do enjoy you will not have to ask somebody else to help you. Having started to read again you may find that you feel like studying. Perhaps you would enjoy doing a short story or journalism course or learn another language using a Linguaphone course or going to an adult education centre. I heard of one woman of over sixty with MS who was doing a course with the Open University; I am hoping to go back to university next year to do a course in creative writing.

If your hands are still mobile you may want to develop other skills such as dressmaking, tailoring, macramé work or lampshade-making. These are only a few of the vast number of courses available at most adult education centres. You must choose the things that you really want to do. This is one of the areas where the problem of having MS with less mobility and increasing fatigue can be turned by you into an opportunity to do some of the things that you once thought would be interesting but never had the time to do.

Chapter 8   Acceptance of MS

Acceptance of MS is difficult to think or write about because it is not a finite act. In 1978, two years after I was diagnosed as having MS, I could have said and believed it to be true, that I had accepted the diagnosis; but I have learned since that real acceptance is ongoing. Perhaps others are more clear-thinking and clear-feeling and acceptance is for them a once-only process.

When the diagnosis was first made I was so shocked that it did not mean anything. After the car crash, when I stayed home and rested, I remember feeling quite stunned about the diagnosis of MS and with a very real sense of loss. The only time that I had had this feeling before was when my father, of whom I was very fond, died.

The diagnosis of any chronic and incurable disease such as MS can have the same effects as a bereavement. The first phase is described as one of shock and bewilderment, denial that anything has happened and a complete failure to realize its significance. I know that during the first weeks I felt numb and lived each day in a mechanical sort of way. It was fortunate for me that the children were living at home and I could continue through the motions of getting breakfast, seeing that they left in time to catch the school bus, pottering about the house, doing a few chores and getting a meal ready for their return in the evening.

This initial stage of shock and bewilderment is followed, in bereavement, by a sense of realization of the loss with either open expressions of grief or outbursts of anger about what has happened. At some point I did realize that something physical had happened to my body that would not go away and over which I had no control or perhaps limited control and I experienced feelings of revulsion about my body. In the past year I have wondered if those strong negative feelings about the body may play some part in the development of MS and the onset of relapses and I shall be writing more about this at the end of this book. In my most recent relapse two years ago I felt intense anger with my body which had let me down when I needed it so badly. Many people experience anger about the way in which the diagnosis is made or the many delays before it is made. They may have had a diagnosis of neurosis previously and feel that if only the correct diagnosis had been made earlier the outlook might have been different. I do not believe that for me an earlier diagnosis would have made much difference and it might have prevented me from doing many things which I am glad that I have done.

The third stage of a reaction to bereavement may be apathy and certainly there was for me ten years ago and times in the past two years when it has seemed too much effort to make positive decisions. It has been easier to sit back and in some ways allow myself to be overtaken by events. This could have happened in a rather child-like way as though I had no real control over my life or the events which change it.

The fourth and final stage of bereavement has been described as one of readjustment, rehabilitation and acceptance. Of course, not all reactions to bereavement run such a straightforward course and not all of them end in acceptance. It is all too easy for the reaction to get held up at the stage of anger and then the future will be bleak and unhappy for the patient and his relatives. In 1976 I made a mental balance sheet of what I had lost and what I still had to my credit. I had to do a great deal of mental spring-cleaning and sort out those things in my life which were of real importance and jettison some undertakings and ambitions which were of less value. I thought that I might have lost longevity but hoped that I should be around for another ten years to see my family through to independence. My recent relapse was just ten years later and at one low point I felt that I had been the loser in a bargain with destiny!

The thought of losing my mobility did not worry me very much in 1976. I had been a bookworm since my early years and there had always been a collection of books around waiting to be read. Less time spent rushing around and more time spent quietly reading could be a welcome change. However, during past months I have cared more and have done everything possible to keep my mobility.

Ten years ago my family had to come first and I knew that in putting them first I had to be very careful to steer away from all thoughts of

77

martyrdom. I have realized that one must learn to be 'constructively' selfish so that the children need never feel guilty in the proper pursuit of their own interests. I also had to learn to say 'no' when asked to take on new commitments – and I have still not learnt that one! Over the years, I have found that there is a narrow margin between restriction of activity, which is good, and hibernation, which is bad and can be destructive of self and even of family. I also had to do a physical spring-clean and clear-up because I found that life was simpler and less tiring if everything was kept in an orderly way. Tidiness was never one of my virtues and it still is not! There never seems to be time to clear up after finishing one job and then there is even less time for the next job after wasting time looking for the 'tools' not put away after the first job and lost in the chaos!

It takes a long time and a lot of self-descipline to learn to achieve the things that are possible rather than habitually failing to achieve those that are impossible. The difference between the two will result either in growing happiness and a renewed sense of fulfilment or repeated frustration and despair. Some would say 'one must learn to fight an illness such as MS.' I would agree with this if a fighting attitude is used in a constructive way towards rebuilding a future and surviving to the best of one's ability. But I have seen a fighting spirit used in the wrong way that has antagonized doctors, family and friends and led to much bitterness and the disruption of valuable relationships. Will-power and a fighting spirit can probably do little to control the disease but if used rightly can help to make the best use of mental and remaining physical powers.

Ten years ago when I started going back to work I was appalled at how tired I got and I was frequently, in my teenage son's word, 'knackered'. I curtailed all my interests apart from doing some journalism to which I was already committed; but as the weeks passed my condition did not improve. In fact the fatigue increased and I was frequently irritable with my family.

All of us who are independent by nature hate to admit that we can no longer do everything for ourselves and we need to come to terms with the fact that we are going to need help. Martyrdom is not a socially attractive characteristic; it is so much better to swallow our pride and accept help with gratitude. Ten years later I had to relearn

78

that lesson with difficulty. I finally accepted the offer of an Orange Badge for my car but at first would stay at home rather than use it. Pride is a poor aid to survival and some of us are remarkably slow to learn that lesson!

During the past two years I have had to do an even more extensive spring-clean. This has included giving up all clinical medicine, becoming more organized as a writer and accepting a lifestyle needing less money. Making a final decision to give up medicine was difficult but my health has greatly improved since I did it. After I knew the 'arithmetic' of early retirement it was clear that I had to balance more money against more time and better health. It was obvious that struggling on for another six years to get a better pension could mean either repeated spells off work or a long struggle with diminishing mobility and increasing fatigue. I had a great sense of relief as soon as I had made the decision to give up medicine.

If you are open about the diagnosis of MS from the time that you are told, I think that it does help you to accept help. I know that some people prefer to keep the diagnosis to themselves, or share it with only the closest friends. For them this may be right but I have had letters from those who at first kept the illness a secret and later when the signs of MS were difficult to hide and they badly needed help could not bring themselves to speak to friends or neighbours and found themselves becoming depressed recluses. I decided early to be open about it and certainly this was a better way for me.

In 1976 we lived in a small and remote community and curiosity is a normal part of village life! You can either look on it as uninvited and unwelcome invasion of your privacy or see it as I did as natural interest in what is happening to other people in the same small community. I realize now that one of the major problems in talking about the diagnosis of MS is the threatening nature of the disease. It is widely known to have the potential power of crippling, causing incontinence and upsetting speech; but it is not as generally known that for the majority of people it is a much milder disease. Only one in five patients will ever need a wheelchair.

After the diagnosis was made I was particularly encouraged to hear about other people with MS who had done well and how much their determination helped. I did not know if determination really helped but it certainly spurred me on to do everything possible to help myself. A writer friend suggested that I should keep a detailed diary because being at the same time a patient, a medical practitioner and a journalist, it might be of use later in my medical or writing work. It certainly helped a lot at the time to keep that diary and once I had written about a problem it often seemed more manageable. I confess that the diary was kept very much more regularly in the bad times than in the good and even after ten years I do not have the courage to read it all. Some of it was too painful to be reread and I can remember as much as I need to without reminding myself of the things written during the darkest times.

I found that the telephone was a mixed blessing. Most phone calls were marvellous and very welcome and cheering. I had my favourite callers who somehow seemed to phone at just the right moment and have the right thing to say. I found on several occasions that you can not 'read' a telephone call again at your leisure. I found that letters could be of greater help because they were more enduring. Sometimes I would read and reread them and they never left me with the rather lost feeling that I sometimes felt after a telephone call. Perhaps at a time of shock and insecurity the physical presence of paper and writing is one of greater comfort than the ephemeral nature of another voice however pleasant at the time. I would exclude one special call from that generalization. During my first week when I was confined to the house and feeling very isolated and vulnerable a friend phoned and said casually that there was a phone by her bed and if I ever felt like a chat during the night she would be there. That meant a lot to me at the time and probably far more than she ever knew. Sadly she died five years ago but I shall always remember her with affection and respect.

During my recent relapse I became aware that it is different and in many ways easier to live in a city with many friends and acquaintances close at hand.

I found ten years ago and again now that visitors are a great delight. At the time when my legs were least predictable I preferred friends to drop in rather than being invited or asking me in advance if it would be convenient. This is probably a personal idiosyncracy but I found my fatigue so variable that I felt upset if I was expecting somebody and then felt too tired to be cheerful. If the caller was unexpected it seemed more excusable to be tired or depressed.

The world is so short of listeners and you do have time when not well to listen to other people's problems and think how they can best be helped. Learning to live with illness includes learning to use your own problems constructively in order to be more outgoing and helpful to others. Self-centredness and self-pity bring you nothing but regrets, isolation and depression. You do have to learn to look outwards rather than inwards and learn to meet people in their lives rather than trying to bring them into yours; this is particularly important at a time when you may not be finding your life a happy one. Learn to listen; get to know people better; find out what makes them happy and try to understand their problems.

All the help your friends give you, whether it is letters, visits, lifts in cars or just chats on the phone help to make you feel a person rather than just a disabled non-person. When you know that you have a potentially disabling disease your feelings about yourself can become so negative. Your friends can help you recognize that you are still the same 'you' and this can be a help in the process of getting back to wholeness. I now believe that many and perhaps the majority of patients with MS have not started with too good an image of themselves even before the bad effects of MS have further lowered their self-esteem.

Getting through the bad patches

MS by its very nature is unpredictable and there cannot be many people with it who do not have to come to terms with the bad patches. I find this unpredictability one of the most difficult things about learning to live with MS. The unexpectedness of these patches makes them more upsetting and much more frightening. One woman described herself as quite different when she was exhausted and knew she was no longer the woman her husband had married. She was no longer able to apologize when the bad patch was over although she knew clearly that she had been a fiend to her family. She felt that she was not responsible for her behaviour and also knew quite certainly that it would happen again.

I used to believe that bad patches were entirely unpredictable but I have come to learn that I usually bring them on myself. Sometimes stresses are unavoidable but there are times when I could have avoided fatigue by weeding out some unnecessary activities or by sorting out my priorities. The bad patch can be a few days of excessive fatigue when it is difficult to get through one's usual work, or it can last longer and as well as fatigue there is a recurrence or increase in old physical symptoms. This does not necessarily mean that the disease has become active again; and there is no good explanation for this variability in symptoms from day to day or even from hour to hour. After the bad patch has passed the chances are that the symptoms will clear up again: a weak leg will be less weak, difficult speech will be less difficult, uncomfortable or painful spasms in your legs may go and blurred vision will to a certain extent improve again.

Sometimes a bad patch can be a relapse in the disease when new symptoms may occur or old symptoms get worse and recovery be less complete. A serious relapse must be managed and treated as an acute episode in the illness and medical help will be necessary.

I think the only way of preventing some of these distressing times is by a greater understanding of yourself, your stresses, your stamina and early signs of fatigue. It all sounds so simple but I know that I am not alone in finding this understanding of myself to be a difficult skill to acquire. If you are feeling well you will naturally want to forget about having anything wrong with you. You may also have the urge to cram into your life all you possibly can while you are feeling well. The biggest incentive for me to try and learn to live at a more moderate pace is that in the end I achieve more of what I want to do if I carry on at a snail's pace rather than keep having to stop if I do spurts like a hare and then have weeks when I can do very little indeed.

Many people with MS find that they have long spells when they really do seem to have far more energy, and are less prone to fatigue and at times like these it is normal and natural to forget about the illness and get on with life with all its opportunities. I managed to do this for five years before my most recent relapse. Some people may remain on a non-animal-fat diet or other diet however well they are, but others will carry on without any controls or restrictions. They may get away with it for years and there is no evidence to show that they would have been better or postponed a relapse longer if they had kept to some sort of regime. Other people have phases of being very much more vulnerable to fatigue, either over a limited time or over many years; and for these people there are one or two possibilities that may make the smooth periods more on a level with the rough ones.

Fatigue and exhaustion should be avoided but it is difficult for many of us to ration our activity and also our output of emotional energy. The greatest risk is when I feel fittest and am sure that I can manage anything. I know that for many, as for me, it goes against the grain to fail to do the things that I have undertaken; but priorities need to be re-examined and possibly changed. From being one who regularly burnt the midnight oil I find that I am now far better if I am in bed by 10 p.m. or earlier, as often as I am able. It is said that you are unable to store sleep like charging a battery, but from my experience it is quite possible to 'bank' some energy by more rest and sleep before undertaking anything that will be particularly tiring.

It is difficult to learn to live a relaxed life with resolution of emotional conflicts as they occur rather than ignoring them and letting them build up. It can be especially difficult if you live in a household of children including teenagers. Any type of mental organization, from contemplative prayer to transcendental meditation may help and I shall write about some ways which I have found helpful at the end of this book. I feel sure that a daily rhythm of physical, mental and spiritual routines helps towards a more balanced way of living.

If, or much more probably, when, you run into a bad patch while trying to live sensibly I can only suggest some ideas that may be helpful. If you are able to 'switch off' and abandon daily chores for a short while it will be best. It might be possible to stay with a good friend for a few days if it is difficult to get any real rest at home. When we were living in Scotland I knew one lovely quiet country inn, not too far away, where I was welcomed and found the sort of peace, hospitality and indeed spoiling, which for me was healing. In a matter of hours my fatigue began to lift and I sometimes used to wish that I had the time and money to go there for a long weekend every month!

Perhaps if your children are older you will be able to have a day or two in bed from time to time if you are very tired. I used to keep a plentiful supply of dried and frozen food in the house, to cater for such times. My own family were good and would cope with house and animals while I had a day in bed. If I am going through a more prolonged bad spell, I can help myself by staying in bed later in the morning. At the moment I take a thermos of coffee to bed with me and drink it in the morning while I lie and write in bed.

I think it is especially important to keep to a disciplined way of life through the bad patches. It is much easier for me to write this than do it myself! There have been times recently when I have been advised by a friend to go and read my own book on MS and take note of what it says! It is so easy to feel that one needs comfort and so cheat about diet, put on weight, not bother about taking any exercise because you feel tired. None of these things in themselves may make much difference but the negative attitude of not caring is self-destructive and not helpful in speeding recovery.

It is difficult to remain outward-looking when literally shut in your house with your own fatigue and possibly unhappy thoughts. It is important never to give up hope however bad the patch or however long it lasts. I do know how impossible it is at times to keep even a glimmer of hope but surprising things can and do happen. Sometimes they are small things; but as long as hope remains alive a small thing can mean a great deal.

Chapter 9 MS and the Family

The question of telling the patient or not telling the patient when MS is first considered a probability is an essential part of the problem of MS and family relationships. It is, perhaps, surprising that communications about MS produce such a minefield of problems. I believe that this is because MS is such a variable disease and is so totally unpredictable. I also believe that the public image of MS must change before a more intelligent and sensitive approach can be made towards introducing the family to the idea that one of its members has MS. Perhaps we need to consider the following points.

1 Fewer than one in five of all people who are diagnosed as having MS will ever be seriously paralysed or need a wheelchair.

2 An unknown and possibly large number of people have symptoms suggestive of MS at some point in their lives but never develop any further problems attributable to MS.

3 The present public image of MS is of terrible tragedies of young people being struck down in their prime. Such tragedies do occur, and at the time of writing this book we are all aware of the tragically early death of the cellist Jacqueline du Pré; but these tragedies are exceptional. The majority of people with MS are handicapped to a certain degree but many not seriously so. If the public image was of such a disease there would not be the same problems in communication between doctor and patients; but because the spectres of wheelchairs, paralysis and incontinence loom as soon as MS is mentioned it is natural that there should be such a dread. It does not help those in the majority with a benign form of MS to feel overshadowed by this spectre lurking in the background. The image of MS must be changed if families are to get better help.

4 MS must not become a new member of the family. It has to be assimilated into the existing family structure. It is a disease of the CNS and can be a very nasty disease but not for the majority of patients.

5 Every problem that a person with MS has is not necessarily attributable to MS. MS must not become a scapegoat. Perhaps the person with MS is being thoroughly difficult and bad-tempered. Any disease, including MS, is unpleasant but it must not be allowed to intrude into and take over every facet of family life.

It is important that there should be as much honesty about the diagnosis as possible, but there can only be honesty if it is realized by everybody concerned, doctor, patient and relatives, that MS can be a very mild disease as well as a very nasty and crippling one. I believe that it is the unpredictability of MS that makes honesty so difficult and can so easily build a lack of trust and a lot of anger into its diagnosis and management. If it can be accepted that MS can be a mild disease, positive steps can be taken towards achieving better physical health and greater emotional stability for the patient and relatives.

Honesty about the variability of the disease is the first requisite for good family communication. It is important that the patient should be encouraged to do as much as possible within the limits of fatigue. MS must not become the family ghost but controlled and lived with as amicably as possible. I think that if such attitudes could prevail fewer marriages and partnerships would break up. I have sometimes seen MS being wielded in a family a little like Alice in Wonderland used the flamingo as a croquet stick. MS must not be used as any sort of weapon.

When any chronic or severe illness affects one member of a married couple the result can either be a bonding process or a disrupting one. Probably this depends on the maturity of the characters involved and the depth of mutual regard and affection which they can bring to, and share in dealing with, the problem. False courage, bravado and inopportune sympathy, demanding behaviour and childish ways all tend to disrupt the relationship. In my own marriage the physical distance between us at the time of my diagnosis and the impossibility of spending much time together and probably my own over-defensiveness all combined to act as disrupting forces. In a close marriage it is impossible to hide deep feelings, fears of disability or death and apprehensions about the future. If they can be shared, much emotional isolation can be avoided and there is a greater chance that the marriage will be strengthened rather than weakened.

Open and honest discussion may be needed about money, for when either a husband or wife is disabled, the amount of effective money for the use of the family inevitably drops. If the husband is unable to work, a disability pension, possibly other insurances, and savings are unlikely to be as great as his original income. The wife may not be able to go out to work for many hours a day to supplement the family income because she will be needed at home to help her husband and cope with the daily chores. If the wife is disabled with MS it is unlikely that the state financial help will recompense the family for the extra expense incurred in replacing the lost work of a wife and mother. Help will be needed for cooking, cleaning and possibly caring for children as well as for the disabled mother. In addition, the husband may find that he has to refuse promotion or to take time off work to cope with many everyday problems with which his wife would previously have coped.

This may be the time to think about your house. Is it in a suitable place or one that is very isolated? Can it be adapted for a disabled person if this should be necessary in the future? Does the smooth running of the home depend on such expensive items as two cars? That may have been fine while there was plenty of money coming in but could be a totally unnecessary burden if there is likely to be less money. It is practical matters such as these that need to be discussed openly. The problems will not go away if they are not talked about. It could also be the right time to think about more modern gadgets in the kitchen to reduce work. Help may be available for such updating of a kitchen from statutory or voluntary sources.

Should children be told about a sick parent, and if they are told how much should they be told and when? It is very difficult to generalize with such a complicated problem. Very small children may be unaware of the family difficulties as long as their physical and emotional needs are attended to by an effective mother substitute. At any age older than this I think there is a far greater danger in under- rather than over-estimating the understanding of children. If they are not told about an illness such as MS their suffering and their sense of exclusion may be much greater than if they are told gently, and progressively kept informed about the illness. It is all-important that their questions should be answered honestly and as fully as they require. Obviously this needs a subtlety of judgement which parents may lack. It is probably more difficult to tell adolescent children than to tell younger children. Adolescence is a vulnerable time when feelings both negative and positive may be running high between parents and offspring. I think there are few families who can honestly say there are no emotional crises during these years. What is going to be the effect on an adolescent of being told that a parent has a possibly progressive and incurable disease such as MS?

I think the same sort of approach should be used in telling the adolescent as in telling the patient. Honesty is paramount but optimism comes a close second. MS is not a death sentence or even a sentence of severe disability; rather is it a diagnosis that needs some thought and considerable adaptation of lifestyle. If this can be explained sensibly and sensitively to an adolescent, the expectation of excessive fatigue on the part of the patient and the consequent demands for help will not be such a problem. Indeed the demands can be another example of problems becoming opportunities.

Is it wrong that children or young people should be forced into situations like this before one believes they are ready to understand the harder facts of life? Obviously the answer depends on the young people concerned, the family as a unit and the strength of the individual bonds within the family. Of course they forget, are careless, thoughtless and occasionally utterly callous, but that is how it should be. Yet underneath this natural behaviour of adolescents towards their middle-aged parents I knew that mine had an unusual protectiveness which might only be shown by a push away from the kitchen sink and a command to go and have an early bath and not take all the hot water.

It is as necessary for a parent with MS to be optimistic with her children as for a doctor to be optimistic with his patient with MS. There is no point in pondering about a bleak future; it is much more important to concentrate on the possibilities of today. It is also important that a parent should at no time blackmail children with her illness. I know from bitter personal experience that this can all too easily happen and at the time be done unwittingly. You must be extremely honest with yourself about your motives and never let personal gain, through your disability or possibility of future disability, influence your actions or attitudes towards your family.

Chapter 10   Sexuality and MS

Pregnancy, contraception and sexual problems can all appear to be conundrums when associated with MS; but it is very difficult to disentangle the problems which can be firmly attributed to MS and those which would have happened to that particular person in any case. The dividing line between the problems of the person who happens to have MS and its effects on that person are intertwined. Therefore, my ideas are individual and none of them may be applicable to you. Each person is unique and you will need individual counselling for your particular problem. All I can do here is to make you more aware of yourself and your needs, give a few generalizations about sexuality and its problems when associated with MS and point you towards places and people where you may be able to find the sort of help you need at the moment.

Sexual problems for the male

Impotence and problems with ejaculation do occur in males with MS, but not necessarily the result of it. They can and do occur with other diseases of the nervous system, in other physical and mental diseases without any physical damage to the CNS and sometimes in men who are apparently fit. It is all too easy for someone to tell you that any sexual problem is caused by MS. Impotence could equally well be caused because you have developed a rather hostile relationship with your partner. This must be stressed because it makes a lot of difference to the sort of help that will be of benefit. If the impotence, or any other problem with ejaculation is associated with a problem in the relationship it may well be curable if the relationship can be sorted out.

It is of paramount importance that the patient with MS should be the one who is asking for help with a sexual problem and not the partner or medical attendant who feels that he should be helped. The patient may not want to have a sexual relationship and therefore may not want help in maintaining one. The help of a medically qualified and psycho-sexually trained counsellor may be vital. It is possible that a man is impotent because of damage to the nervous tissue in his spinal cord; but it is more likely that he has become impotent because of his own inner rage about his changed body and the damage to himself and to his relationship. Help may be needed with the relationship rather than with just having sex or getting physical help with a prosthesis. Such help may be inopportune and insensitive. The impotent man may need space to express his anger rather than any sympathy or supportive type of counselling. Release of anger and its subsequent acceptance with a deeper understanding of all the problems can mean reconciliation within and around the patient.

If a man is having nocturnal erections it can be assumed that the nervous connections controlling erections are intact and some sort of skilled counselling could help. But it must be stressed that any possi-bility of help is conditional on the patient wanting and asking for it.

Sexual problems in women

A woman's sexual problems, as in men with MS, are more likely to be associated with problems in the relationship than caused by physical damage to the CNS.

A woman who is physically tired and emotionally drained may have problems with lubrication of the vagina and reaching orgasm, whether or not she has MS. She will need help with her own physical and mental state and with her relationship. When those facets of her life are sorted out her sexual problems may also be resolved. She may benefit from treatment from a skilled psychosexual counsellor. Again it must be stressed that she must want such help. If she has no motivation to change her attitudes to herself and her partner and prefers to blame MS for anything that has gone wrong, time spent with a counsellor will be wasted.

Contraception

There is no evidence that any particular form of contraception is best for or contra-indicated for a patient with MS. The choice of contraception should be discussed with a doctor who is experienced in family planning and all the problems associated with MS and reproduction can then be talked about openly and with both partners present. The following points about contraception must be considered, and these are the same as for any other couple about to start a sexual relationship.

1 The acceptability to both partners.

2 The need for total reliability if pregnancy is not wanted.

3 Any particular risk factors for avoiding the combined oral contraceptive (COC) such as high blood pressure or a deep-vein thrombosis. MS by itself is not a contra-indication for the COC.

4 Any risk factors for the intra-uterine device (IUD) such as a previous ectopic pregnancy or pelvic inflammatory disease.

The only problems which may be particular to patients with MS are a difficulty with insertion of a cap or use of a condom because of clumsy hands. It may be acceptable to both partners that the one who does not have MS is responsible for the use of a barrier method, but that depends on the individuals and not only on clumsy hands.

Pregnancy

In the past, that is until the 1950s, pregnancy was regarded as a high-risk factor for a woman with MS and there is probably a slightly greater risk of a relapse occurring during the first three months after delivery. There is no firm evidence that pregnancy does make MS worse, however, and it is up to each couple to make their own decision. Obviously if the woman is in relapse, pregnancy should be delayed or if the future of either partner is particularly vulnerable pregnancy may be better avoided long-term. A woman who has MS should not be given steroids during her pregnancy and should avoid having a spinal anaesthetic during her delivery. She should also have physical help and emotional support during the months after delivery; but this could be said about many mothers-to-be and most first-time mothers. A survey published in an American medical journal, *Neurology*, in 1986 reported that 178 mothers with MS had no long-term worsening of the disease after childbirth compared with the control group of women with MS who did not have a pregnancy.

Can MS be inherited by a child?

There is no evidence of any recognizable pattern of inheritance as with some other diseases, but there is a slightly increased incidence of MS among the children of parents who have MS. This increased susceptibility could be due to a similar background and place of upbringing rather than to an inherited genetic pattern.

Chapter 11   MS and Work

Occupation has a vital role to play in keeping up morale in any illness and particularly in a chronic and unpredictable illness such as MS. It is realistic and not pessimistic to make an early assessment of the work you are doing now and hope to do in the future. I now believe that this is particularly important because it could be the stresses in living that precipitate the onset and relapses in MS. Therefore, an intelligent assessment of work by the patient with possibly some professional help may not only be wise for the present but also for the future of the patient and his family. It is always better to make long-term plans while in a state of calm rather than being forced into making a decision at a time of crisis. The MS Society knows that more people with MS have to give up work because of fatigue than disablement. It is possible that the fatigue is a sign of the inner stresses of the person with MS. An honest and critical appraisal of what work is doing to the person may make an important contribution to a long remission in the disease and a benign outcome.

If you are physically able to manage the job you are doing when MS is diagnosed it is so easy, especially if you have a good boss, just to keep on going in the same old way ignoring fatigue and not thinking about the future. A sort of let's grit our teeth, keep a stiff upper lip and carry on mentality. Perhaps for some people with especially strong ostrich tendencies this may be the only way, and for others this approach may give them more peace of mind and confidence for the future.

At the time of my last relapse, two years ago, I had a good boss and soon after I had gone off sick he telephoned to reassure me that my job would be kept open for me, adding that the worst that could happen to me would be confinement to a wheelchair and he felt sure that conditions at work could be adapted to my needs. At that time it was immensely reassuring to hear this; but gradually over the next months I realized that going back to the same job would mean more ill health, relapses in my MS and chronic fatigue. The stresses at work had contributed to my relapse and to go back into them with the further complication of increased physical handicap was not going to help me. Having a close and critical look at myself helped me to make decisions about my own future with or without relapses in MS. And I think this sort of cool appraisal needs to be made for each person who develops MS.

There is never going to be a perfect way of living and working. More congenial work with greater job satisfaction and fewer stresses may mean less money or job security; but these problems may be worth it if in the long-term there will be better health and improved family relationships. I had to make a sort of balance sheet of the advantages and disadvantages of giving up work. The main advantages for me in giving up work were gaining control over my time and energy, more time at home and the health benefits of release from the stresses at work about which I could do nothing. The disadvantages were less money, much less pension, a loss of status, the possibility of isolation and the loss of friends at work. Obviously this sort of profit-and-loss account would not be relevant for someone with young children to bring up, but the ideas of cool appraisal, the acceptance of outside help in decision-making and in the end accepting responsibility for one's own future are the same for any patient. Nobody knows what the future holds but the more you can feel in control of what you are choosing to do, the more likely you are to have a long remission and possibly stay well for many years. For me it has worked well; and many of the disadvantages that I foresaw have not happened. Certainly I have very much less money but I can adapt to that and I rejoice in greater freedom in the use of my time, energy and abilities.

Only you as the patient can make the final decision about work but a real understanding of yourself is most important before you can make a wise and informed decision. Perhaps you are young, intelligent and ambitious. You see your future as a doctor, lawyer or businessman. You should stop and consider if you are really doing what you think is best for you or being driven by foolish ambition and greed. Examinations are stressful and excessive responsibility can precipitate relapses.

If you want to get to the top in any profession you have to work long hours and often under great physical and mental pressure. If MS is diagnosed early in your career it may be better for your health to choose a steady and less competitive line in your chosen career. For instance, in medicine it would probably be better to aim at a speciality with fewer emotional demands and less night work. It may also be worth considering a speciality where it may be possible at times to do part-time work.

If you have any creative talents it is a good idea to think seriously about developing them while you are still physically well. You may say it is quite pointless because you only daub and could not possibly paint, or that you love writing letters but could not possibly write anything that could be published. I think there are two fallacies here. The first is that creative hobbies do not have to be looked on as potentially lucrative now or later. It is far more important for you as a person to develop something that is pleasurable for you and gives you a sense of achievement. The second fallacy is that hobbies at which you feel only moderately competent could not possibly be sources of income now or later. This is just not true. If your hands are still nimble there is always a demand for simple dress-making, mending or alterations. So many people are terrified of doing even the simplest alteration to a dress but are quite prepared to pay somebody else to do it.

A breadwinner or a potential breadwinner for the family should think early about future employment which will bring a sense of satisfaction as well as providing adequate money for any dependents. In the ten years since I wrote my first book on MS, the whole complexion of employment has changed and it is now more difficult to have freedom of choice, but my ideas have also changed about how much money is sufficient for my needs and sufficiency now seems to me a most important word. Some men and women will decide to go to part-time day or evening classes to learn a new skill such as secretarial work or word-processing or computer-programming. Some may think it would be an opportune moment to do a university degree either through the Open University or as an external student of a university. The balance has to be understood between ridiculous pushing of yourself and finding new interests and real fulfilment.

Journalism can be a useful and paying hobby or possibly even a main employment. Freelance journalism can be quite lucrative but is unlikely to provide a good and steady income unless you are very fortunate. If you feel like trying freelance journalism, short-story writing or writing plays for radio or television it can be a good idea to do a correspondence course to get you started. I have had dealings with the London School of Journalism and found them reliable, responsible and constructive in their help. It is worth investing in a light electronic typewriter early in any writing activity and even a few lessons in typing can be helpful. A word processor is now another useful gadget. It is much lighter to use than a conventional typewriter although it can take some getting used to. I found that the instruction manual of 400 pages of gobbledegook quite impossible to follow, but a weekend course at a local adult education college gave me the courage to get on and have a go.

You will gain if you can live near your work because you can then avoid much of the fatigue and frustration of travelling. It is better to be honest with your workmates about MS, but present a picture of MS as it really is and not as it is so often portrayed publicly. Most people are very willing to help if they know how and why help is needed. It is essential that your employer and foreman, if you have one, should know about any physical problems you have because necessary adaptations to tools or physical facilities can then be made.

Chapter 12   Management of Special Problems

There are many special problems for patients with MS; and here I shall only be writing about some of the ones found most often. Whatever problem you are having at the moment will, of course, be 'special' for you and you must not feel that it is unimportant because it is not discussed here. Possibly the MS Society or ARMS will be able to help you or give you some information about where help could be found.

Muscle spasms

Many people with MS are troubled with muscle spasms and muscle twitching. They may be relatively minor and without pain; or they can be part of a general and sometimes painful increase in the 'tone' of muscles, which may be called spasticity. I have found that the backs of my thighs are liable to go into spasm when I am sitting on a soft chair or soft car seat and in bed at night if I am particularly tired either physically or mentally. It is not usually painful but is an unpleasant feeling and is sufficiently disturbing to stop me from sleeping soundly. I have found, by a process of trial and error, that the most effective way of stopping the spasm is by exercising and strengthening the 'antagonists'. The antagonists of a muscle are those that work in the opposite direction: thus if the muscles at the back of the thigh are in spasm, and those are the ones that are often troublesome, straight leg-raising which will make the muscles on the front of the thigh work hard will stop the spasm. In a car, where straight leg-raising is not feasible, lifting the thigh off the seat while pressing down on the knee may give relief from the spasm. You may, however, be able to find a more effective way for yourself.

Severe spasm or spasticity, caused by an increased tone in the affected muscles, occurs in more severe MS and it is the result of the demyelination of motor nerves. It can be relieved to some extent by diazepam or more effectively by baclofen.

I have discovered during the past two years that different forms of meditation and contemplation have helped my own muscle tightness and spasm and I shall write more about this in Part Three.

Pain

It used to be said that MS did not cause pain but in recent years it has been accepted that MS can and does cause pain which can be difficult to treat by orthodox medical methods of pain relief. The management of pain in MS can be a relatively simple matter if the pain is caused by an identifiable lesion such as optic neuritis or trigeminal neuralgia. The pain of optic neuritis, which can be a very sharp pain made worse by moving the eyes or pressing on the eyeballs, can usually be relieved by steroids. The pain of trigeminal neuralgia, which can be very severe and make the patient depressed, can usually be helped by Tegretol. The depression, which can be associated with severe pain, may be helped by antidepressant therapy, which may at the same time help the pain.

If pain cannot be relieved by the treatment of your general practitioner or neurologist you may be referred to a special pain-relief clinic. These clinics are now established throughout the UK.

Bladder and bowel problems

The process of passing urine and the nerve supply to the bladder are complicated. The bladder wall is made of smooth muscle, that is muscle not under the control of a person's will, and the muscle round the sphincter at the exit from the bladder which is partly under conscious control. Normally, as the bladder fills with urine the bladder wall stretches and the muscle at the sphincter remains contracted. When the bladder has collected between 300 and 500mls of urine the feeling of wanting to pass urine will be experienced, but the passage of the urine can be voluntarily inhibited until it is convenient to urinate. When it is convenient the brain sends messages via the spinal cord, the muscle of the bladder contracts and at the same time the muscle of the sphincter relaxes and the bladder can then empty itself completely.

Various problems can occur in MS depending on the site where demyelination and plaque formation have occurred in the CNS. In the first group of problems control of the bladder may be damaged by a plaque of demyelination so that, in the same way as the knee jerk may become more vigorous in MS, the bladder becomes too sensitive to smaller-than-normal amounts of urine and this causes the problems of urgency, frequency, nocturia, reflex incontinence and enuresis. A hyperexcitable bladder is also often associated with impaired emptying. An increase in muscle tone can also cause simultaneous contraction of the muscles of the bladder and sphincter with difficulties in passing urine.

Less often in MS the muscles of the bladder can become sluggish (in the same way as a knee jerk may be diminished in MS) and this can cause hesitancy, overflow incontinence, retention of urine, urgency, frequency and nocturia. Incomplete emptying of the bladder from any cause makes it more likely that the urine will be infected, causing cystitis, which will mean the frequent and painful passage of urine.

Management of bladder problems

Urgency is very common in MS and can be the only problem in benign forms of the disease. Once the desire to pass urine occurs it can be impossible to prevent the onset of micturition. Regular visits to the toilet, perhaps at half-hour or hourly intervals, will help. I have found that 'disasters' are much more likely to occur when I am near the toilet, for instance while I am putting my key in the front-door lock. If, at that moment, I can deliberately distance my thoughts from my bladder, disasters are much less likely. I realize this sounds fanciful and it does take a lot of practice. I do know that it works, although for me it is certainly not 100 per cent successful. One drift from concentration or an anxious thought and disasters can still occur!

More severe problems with the bladder may need skilled assessment at a urodynamic clinic to decide which part of the mechanism of bladder control has gone wrong; and how the problem can best be helped. Problems of incontinence or the inability to pass urine cause very great anxiety and it is important that emotional support and counselling are given as well as any other treatment which is considered necessary.

After assessment of bladder function and identification of where the lesion is in the CNS, management may include the use of a drug such as baclofen to reduce the amount of spasm in the bladder muscle, regular catheterization by the patient or carer, an indwelling catheter or sometimes surgery may relieve the problem. Until incontinence can be controlled the patient will be advised about the use of incontinence pads, the amount of fluid to drink, the care of the perineal skin and possibly the use of urinary antiseptics to prevent urine infection.

Bowel problems

Constipation is a common problem for people with MS. It can be due to a number of causes directly or indirectly caused by the nervous disease. Directly, a sluggish bowel or poor abdominal muscles can be caused by demyelination of nerves. Indirectly, it can be caused by fatigue or immobility both of which will restrict the amount of physical activity.

Constipation can be helped by taking as much physical exercise as possible, increasing fluid intake, increasing fruit, vegetables and bran in the diet, and cutting out all sugar.

Complete loss of control of bowel action is rare in MS, but apparent loss of control can happen if constipation is severe and liquid faeces begin to leak round the faecal masses. It is then necessary to deal with the severe constipation, clear the bowel possibly by enemas and then re-educate the bowel to evacuate regularly again.

Coping with falls

Falling over has been one of my major problems and I know that many other people with MS have found the same. I do not like falling over partly because it hurts; but a much greater problem is the sense of hurt.

I find it upsetting in a much more general way than the results of the physical damage. So far I have not broken a bone but with advancing years and normal thinning of bones this could easily happen. Obviously it would be much better to avoid falls; therefore I have thought hard about why and when I fall.

The reasons for my falls may not, of course, be the same as yours. I have very little feeling in my left foot and a diminished 'muscle joint sense' in both my feet. So my feet do not automatically do the sensible and normal things; in fact sometimes they seem to be deliberately doing totally mad things. I walk with the help of faith and eyesight. If I am walking on rough ground in the country I must watch where my feet are and make adjustments for one or the other getting into mud or a dip in the ground. At the present time, in 1988, you are as likely to find strange dips in the pavement in the centre of London as in the deepest country; possibly that goes for a lot of other cities. It only needs an unexpected hole in the pavement, one foot down a little from its expected position and I go over. Three of my worst falls have been in Baker Street, Charing Cross Road and the Strand. And I have no intention of going all the way round a Monopoly board to test the hardness of the rest of London's well-known streets! Those three have been sufficient.

All those falls happened when I was tired, carrying too much luggage and in one way or another at a time when my mind was a long way from my feet. So what have I learnt that will prevent me, and hopefully you, from falling over?

1 Allow sufficient time to get from A to B. I still hope to cram into a day when I am well as much as I could when twenty years old and healthy. This is stupid and I must try to be more realistic. It is better to miss a train, be late for an appointment because you have travelled carefully and arrived in order than because you fell over and spent time picking up the pieces and feeling too shaken to continue in a tranquil fashion.

2 What about a stick? When my legs are at their worst I must use a stick because otherwise I am too unsteady to walk safely. But when my legs are much improved I prefer not to use a stick. This may be pride but I prefer to think that it is because I do not want to be

labelled. My friends in the MS Society say that this is foolish and I should use a stick at all times. Certainly it might prevent some falls and with a stick in one hand I could not be carrying luggage, shopping, etc. in both hands. There are advantages and disadvantages about using a stick and at different times the balance in favour of using one will change. Only you will know what is wisest for you at any particular time; and you will only know this if you take note of your own body and its needs. Wise decisions are rare treasures for those with MS. This is another example of someone with MS doing something because of pressure from outside. I had to hurry to catch that train, there were too many people around and somebody pushed me, and all the other excuses. It is also another example of being centred in oneself and that being, thinking, living, and walking need to be directed from the centre outwards. It is not good to be perpetually pushed around, literally and metaphorically, by all the pressures on the outside.

Chapter 13   MS and its Mental Effects

MS is a disease or possibly it could be a whole collection of diseases where emotional problems can both be causes and results. During an illness such as MS there is no doubt that you are more liklely to have emotional upsets than when you are in good health, but there seems little doubt that emotional upsets can cause the onset of a relapse or the temporary worsening of symptoms. There are difficulties with fatigue, with adjustments in learning to do less, there are frequently family stresses and there is always a certain measure, variable indeed but recurrent, of personal anxiety.

For each person the situations that lead to fatigue will be different; but for everyone there is the same need for facing up to the problems honestly and for determination in finding solutions. It is very much easier to be philosophical about marital problems, difficult situations at work, adolescent offsprings' love problems and unexpected visitors if one is not already overtired.

It is said that euphoria or undue cheerfulness occurs in MS but I have seldom seen it and have certainly not experienced it myself. I think depression is very much more common and can occur at many stages of the disease. It seems to be common in the early stages after the patient is told the diagnosis and must come to terms with it; and this is probably one of the ways in which MS is like a bereavement. Depression can occur after a good period followed by worsening of symptoms, a bad patch of fatigue or a more serious relapse. I think that some of these times of depression can be shortened, lessened or even avoided by taking enough physical and mental rest. A bad patch of depression which does not lift with time and attention to physical conditions may be treated successfully with antidepressants. Some methods which have helped me are given in the last part of this book.

It is important to come to terms with these spells of depression because they are unnerving and distressing. They do seem to be a part of MS for many people; and if they can be accepted as an inevitable part of MS and usually associated with fatigue, they need not be so overwhelming. They come but they pass and are something that has to be avoided as far as possible but when unavoidable accepted philosophically.

There is no question of fault about getting ill but you do have some responsibility for getting tired, irritable and depressed. There is a question of responsibility for yourself; are you trying to allocate your limited energy in the most sensible way? Are you having a rest during the day? Do you stop doing a job before you are exhausted? And a question for me at the moment: does it really make sense to work until 5a.m. even with a deadline to finish this book? Well, of course, I shall be able to have an early night tomorrow.

I believe now that there is often no clear-cut division between illness that is mental, physical or spiritual. Sadly, orthodox medical practitioners still have to think and work with divisions between physical and mental illness, but ideas are changing and will, I think, continue to change. A psychiatrist can now be the wisest physician because he is more able to look at the whole person than another physician who by his training will be concentrating on one system of the body such as the cardiovascular or nervous system. If one considers the person as a whole it no longer seems as important if a misdiagnosis of MS as a psychiatric disease does occur. And possibly the wise psychiatrist has as much to offer the patient with MS about learning to live with it as does the neurologist.

Dementia is very rare in MS and occurs only late in severe and progressive MS. An inability to concentrate and poor memory are much more likely to be caused by depression or anxiety than by dementia. These symptoms will get better as the underlying mental state is helped. I am sure that many mental states which are attributed to MS can be helped by honest communication with another person. Distress of one sort or another can so easily be covered up by a false jollity, but once dishonest communications have started they can so easily be perpetuated. In the end this can cause confusion and misunderstanding instead of open and honest communication. If I am sad it is better to know that I am sad and be able to share my sadness even with one other person than have to pretend to everybody, including myself, that I am jolly. Dishonesty can only cause greater distress in the long run and more mental confusion.

Counselling offers a multitude of help from giving support and information to treatment for a psychosexual problem. Essentially skilled counselling is a means of helping the person with MS to be able to take his own responsibility for his own body and his future. Both the MS Society and ARMS provide counselling and information about suitable training for would-be counsellors.

Chapter 14   Doctors and MS

If you already have a trusted general practitioner when you are diagnosed as having MS, you will probably not want to change. If you are choosing a doctor, when you already know you have MS, and you are not likely to be moving house soon, you will want to consider the arrangement as a long-term one. You may not need to see him frequently and this will depend not only on the severity of your MS and the occurrence of a relapse but also on your self-sufficiency and your need for encouragement and support. Our domestic circumstances as well as our resilience will affect our need for support.

I think that one of the most important attributes that any doctor, general practitioner or specialist, can have is to be able to talk to you as a person rather than at you as a patient. If your doctor, by the way in which he speaks to you, can make you feel a more whole person he will be giving you a great healing service. The doctor, by his attitude, can minimize or exacerbate our feelings of disability. Most problems in MS are going to be fairly long-standing ones and although the moment will come when you feel you must ask for help, the more reasonable and considerate you are of your doctor's time the more considerate he is likely to be of your problem.

Doctors prefer you to remember the various things you want to ask them rather than producing a 'shopping list' and working through it! And the doctor will also be pleased if you do try to think about the advice he is giving you and act on it once you can see that it is reasonable. Weight reduction comes within this sphere of help.

Other doctors are called consultants or specialists. These doctors have higher qualifications in their chosen speciality. You will be most likely to see a neurologist but there is no particular reason to see a neurologist at regular intervals unless you or he or your GP prefers you to do this.

When a diagnosis of MS is made, the patient and his family may go in one of two directions about treatment. With a little knowledge about MS it may be easy to get into a state of despair and imagine that because there is no cure there is nothing at all to be done. This is more likely to happen without some positive medical direction and encouragement. At the opposite extreme the patient and his relatives may refuse to accept advice but believe that if they try hard enough, travel far enough, and possibly spend enough money, they will find a way for the patient to be 'cured'. There is no point in moving house to be nearer a research centre. You can just as easily follow a sensible regime where you are living at present.

When learning to accept and live with a long-term and variable illness like MS you need a doctor whom you can trust and to whom you can turn at times of real difficulty. On the other hand you must learn to cope with most of your own problems and be responsible for your own decisions. It can be tempting to lean too heavily on your doctor and then be prepared to blame him when things get worse. Doctors can only give advice – they do not usually work miracles.

In the course of my own illness, I believe that in 1976 when the diagnosis of MS was first made the future of our relationship would have been different if my husband and I had seen the London neurologist together. On occasions when the same sort of problem is occurring a joint visit to a wise neurologist can prevent the isolation of the patient who gets walled up with MS and the spouse who feels left out and retaliates by saying that MS is just a flight of the imagination. The resolution of this sort of problem at an early stage can help not only the progress of MS but even more importantly the marital and family relationships.

When the doctor first considers MS a possibility he may believe that the patient should not be told. The first symptom may be blurred vision in one eye or transient tingling in an arm or leg. There may be some signs of MS at that time but it is possible that the disease will not progress or recur. At the first incident it could be a mistake to tell the patient that she has MS because it might cause needless worry and suffering and such a prognosis could even become self-fulfilling. If there was a proven cure it could be very wrong not to tell the patient; but there is no such cure.

At a time of recurrence of symptoms, the problems of telling or not telling get more difficult. What are the patient and relatives thinking? Their fantasies may be much worse than the reality. I am sure that any communication from the doctor to the patient must be the truth but not necessarily the whole truth. If you feel that you want to know the truth it will be partly up to you to make this clear and show yourself able and willing to accept it and cope with the problems. I believe, and have discussed elsewhere, that honesty will be easier when the public image of MS can become more realistic than at present.

Part Three

Chapter 15   Exploring Sickness and Health

Introduction

Perhaps I should describe this part of the book as a jigsaw puzzle with many pieces missing. I am not even too sure what the finished puzzle will look like. I am not academic, or a medical researcher, or trained in psychology, theology or philosophy. However, I shall attempt to write down some of my thoughts and understandings of the past two years about sickness and health and about MS. I am not claiming some new way of curing MS or a short cut to health for all. I believe that the way to any sort of healing or wholeness is essentially an individual one and for much of the time a lonely one. What I shall write will be in the nature of an 'interim' report because I hope that my understanding will continue to grow; and I hope that for some readers this may be of value. I stress that I am writing about my personal understanding of my own experiences during this time and my interpretation of the experiences of other people with MS which they have shared with me. I fully realize that for many and perhaps the majority of general practitioners and neurologists, for many patients with MS and their carers and support groups much of this will be unfamiliar territory, but I hope that a few patients and their doctors may think afresh about physical, psychosomatic and mental illness and the whole field of human disease and health. What I write may apply to all human disease and I emphasize and stress repeatedly that I am not trying to prove that MS is not a physical disease. It is a physical disease of the central nervous system with a known pathology and it is incurable and untreatable.

At the time of writing this book there is growing medical and lay interest in alternative and complementary medicine and also in the movement for holistic medicine. This is therefore an opportune moment to write about my changed understanding of MS which is important not only for the management of this particular disease but more importantly for an understanding of health.

Healing and curing

There is an essential difference between healing and curing with which some readers may be familiar but for the benefit of others I shall try to explain. Curing can be done *by* the doctor or other 'curer' *for* the patient and for some diseases such as cancer the cure can be measured in terms of the survival time of the patient. The doctor is active and the patient passive. To take one example: a patient has cancer of the breast. She is operated on and has chemotherapy and five years later she is alive and without a recurrence of the cancer. She can, therefore, be claimed as a cure. However, if she remains haunted by thoughts of cancer, is recurrently depressed and her marriage has broken up she cannot be thought of as healed. Healing, I believe, must have a large element of patient choice and involvement. In this example the patient is cured but not healed. It is also possible to give an example of a person who is healed but not cured. A peaceful death preceded by family reconciliation can be called healing but clearly death is not a cure in the medical sense. Indeed, death is usually seen as failure by the medical profession. Curing can become the avoidance of death; but healing may be the understanding of joy and love and peace and end in death.

For those people who have severely disabling MS curing could mean being able to walk again but healing might mean the attainment of peace of mind and the ability to make a full contribution to a warm and loving family life. Curing is about the disease and healing about the whole person including the disease. They are not mutually exclusive and sometimes cure can follow healing: but this is not necessarily so.

My responsibility

I do not claim that the ideas expressed here are all original because many of them have come through reading the books of others and also from the talks I have had with many wise people during the past two years; but the responsibility for what I am writing here is mine alone. During these two years of what I can only describe as a fascinating, exciting and at times lonely and terrifying journey of exploration I have had the immense good fortune of an ongoing discussion with a medical friend who is an orthodox general practitioner. At times she has doubted my sanity and the wisdom of pursuing ideas that were denying me the 'comfort' of accepting a physical disease; but her interest has given me the courage to continue my own strange journey.

I could not have written about sickness and health in this way ten years ago when I wrote my first book on MS; all the ideas would have been totally alien to me. Neither could I have written about them two years ago during the early weeks of my most recent relapse because they would have been too painful and out of perspective. I needed time to understand that I have some choice about being sick or healthy. I also had to learn that MS, the disease which I most certainly have, is an integral part of me as a person. It is not some sort of devil within me that can be blamed for all my failures and inadequacies. It would be very nice to have something over which I had no control and that was medically speaking incurable. It could be responsible for everything I did not like about myself and for every problem with which I am unable to cope. I believe now that I do have quite a lot of control over how well or how ill I am.

My physical disease

It might be reasonable for the reader to question whether I really have MS, and I can only reply that two years ago I was ill and had physical signs in my CNS indicative of MS in relapse. I voluntarily surrendered my driving licence while both my feet were numb and my legs too weak to drive a car. Later I had a medical examination to decide if I was fit enough to drive again and my left leg was only just strong enough. I shall need another examination shortly and I doubt if my left leg is now adequately strong to drive a car without automatic transmission. Two years ago I felt exhausted and walking was very difficult. During these two years I have come to feel well but only at the cost of learning many painful lessons and making some difficult choices. I have discovered that my health is not something that can be restored by a doctor or any sort of treatment outside me but it is something over which I have influence if I sincerely wish to be as whole as possible. As with most choices to be made during life I cannot have everything and having chosen health I have had to relinquish many things which I would once have believed of very great importance to me. But it is an exciting journey and one that I want to share as honestly as possible.

My medical orthodoxy

Two years ago I was a fairly orthodox medical practitioner and I believed illness could be subdivided into diseases of the body and mind and could usually be fitted into a diagnostic category. However, if one accepts, as I am beginning to do, that each human is an interlinked whole of body, mind and spirit and that any sickness can affect varying proportions of this indivisible trinity, dis-ease may well not fit a medically acceptable diagnostic category. An indivisible fusion of body, mind and spirit could mean a totally different understanding of sickness and health.

Healing is normal

I now believe that health and a return to health after sickness are the norms for a human. Our cuts heal 'normally' when we have removed any 'foreign bodies', cleaned them up and given them some protection from daily use. Normal healing of a cut will be delayed if the skin edges are far apart and good suturing will accelerate healing; but once favourable conditions have been established the body can get on with its normal process of repair. Our recurrent virus infections, such as colds, measles, mumps and the like, mostly get better without 'treatment' in the orthodox medical sense. A cold usually gets better on its own but its normal resolution may be impaired if a child is living in an atmosphere polluted by cigarette smoke. Normal healing of the cold may then perhaps be delayed by the development of bronchitis

116

and antibiotics will be used; but removal from the smoky atmosphere might have allowed healing from the cold virus without the development of bronchitis. In many diseases, and perhaps many more than we realize at present, the body would heal itself if it could be helped over the obstacle that is preventing the healing. We already know something about the optimum physical conditions for healing to take place; these include treatment of infection, the right sort of diet, the correction of anaemia and any recognizable vitamin deficiencies and perhaps the provision of rest and warmth. We also understand that babies need tender, loving care to thrive and develop normally. We are not so sensitive to such emotional needs in adults, although we are aware of social deprivation and do quite a lot about the manipulation of the social environment.

Obstacles to healing

If we can accept that healing is normal for humans given the right environment then we need to consider the things which may prevent healing. This could be even more important than looking at the pathology of disease when once it is established. Instead of looking for cures or ways of intervention we could start looking at the obstacles to what would be happening normally if those obstacles could be removed or a way found round them.

I would suggest that the first major obstacle is the lack of an honest desire for healing. It is one thing to demand to be made better; but it is a very different thing to decide that one will do everything possible to get better. The one is passive and the other active. 'Of course, everybody wants to get well and nobody would choose to remain ill.' I should most certainly have said that two years ago. I definitely did not want my legs to be so weak that they stopped me doing a job I wanted to do and enjoyed, that provided me with a good income, status as a medical practitioner, security for the rest of my working days and the certainty of a good, index-linked pension at the end of my working life. Why could I possibly have preferred to get ill? Of what possible advantage could it have been to me? And yet looking back now I can see the enormous number of stresses in my life at that point. I know that I did not make a conscious decision to get ill, and when my legs were too weak to get me up the stairs at work I was profoundly distressed about the present and depressed about the future.

A secondary gain from illness?

Two years ago the idea of a secondary gain from illness such as cancer or MS would not have crossed my mind. The first thoughts about such a strange thing were given to me by a retired general practitioner, Ian Pearce, who had become interested in unconventional ways of healing for cancer patients. I saw him about six weeks after I had been off work although he did not normally see people with arthritis or MS because he had no success in helping them.

He did not inquire about my illness or ask why I had come to see him. I could not have told him because I had no idea! He had recently had an operation himself for cancer and he talked about his own illness and his theories about the development of cancer. But the most important part of that talk for me was his idea about the secondary gain from illness. I understood later that there might not only be gain for the patient but also for relatives and professional and voluntary supporters.

I read Ian Pearce's book, *The Gate of Healing*, and found many helpful ideas in it. It is a book written primarily for and about patients with cancer. I do not believe that this book is a blueprint for the healing of cancer or that it could be 'translated' into a book for curing MS. But I certainly found some understanding of health and disease and clues for understanding and accepting myself.

A time for illness?

My last relapse was the worst in my illness. It came at the time when I was, on the one hand doing a tough medical job and for the first time in my professional life using just about all my talents in my work and enjoying it, and on the other hand, trying to cope with increasing family demands. I was enjoying the work but there was no spare time or energy to use for the people around to whom I had a real (as against a professional) commitment.

This was my particular Achilles heel; the dilemma was between doing the things that I believed I was good at, being needed by patients and colleagues and at the same time trying to give to those who were closest to me with seemingly inseparable family ties. I certainly could not see that I might need some space of my own. Neither could I see in November 1985 any sort of priority in the needs of all those making demands on me, or decide which ones I could meet and which I could not.

I must stress that for each person the conflicts will be different and also emphasize that MS is a physical disease. I believe that eventually other diseases will be found to have some sort of conflict at their origin, but that will not be in my lifetime. Conventional medical research looks at what happens after the disease has started; but perhaps one day we shall be looking at the maintenance of real health and the reasons why people fail to heal normally.

The secondary gain from illness can resolve many different sorts of conflict. The dominant and aggressive parent who becomes bound to a wheelchair may resolve many family problems and possibly give a marital partner a new meaning to life after retirement or perhaps after children have left home. I met one MS patient who said freely that having MS was the best thing that had ever happened to him. It released him, as the only boy in the family, from the financial burden of supporting ageing and difficult parents and allowed him to have the sort of social life he had always wanted. It is unlikely that many people could talk as openly about things which might be considered shameful and best not publicized. The person with MS or any other chronic illness is not deliberately using the illness to escape responsibilities but because of the illness the whole pattern of a relationship or relationships within a family will be changed and sometimes for the better.

The secondary gain from illness can prevent the patient's taking any active or self-motivating part in getting better, but at the same time he can still express a desire to be made better, in spite of himself. His family and friends may also be ambivalent about his cure and collude in the maintenance of his illness.

The desire to get better

Healing can only be possible if it is wanted by the patient. In other words you must ask for and be willing to accept help before healing can begin. Insincerity in this desire will mean that healing in its fullness will be impossible. A patient can be cured of an acute appendicitis while remaining completely passive; but with most illnesses of doubtful origin and chronic nature there must be a genuine desire to get better before healing is possible. This may be one of the reasons why doctors make very bad patients. They are not used to asking for or accepting help and believe if they are ill that they can solve the matter for themselves. This may have something to do with their high rates of suicide, alcohol and drug dependence and divorce. It requires a degree of humility to go and ask for help and I think that many doctors including myself, are lacking in this quality. Naturally any patient with a progressive and incurable physical disease would deny wanting to keep his illness. My 'orthodox' medical practitioner friend, who at first thought my ideas about a patient not wanting to lose his MS very eccentric, later told me that she had five patients with MS and has now come to see that each has the 'ability' which is totally at a subconscious level to keep the level of illness that resolves the conflicts around him. But MS is unquestionably a physical illness and I am not implying the possibility of malingering. Perhaps there is also some sort of subconscious choice in other chronic diseases. I am writing about MS because that is the disease that I know from the inside.

The anger that can prevent healing

The wrong use of anger is, I believe, a further reason for failure to return to health. Nobody doubts the amazing power that anger can have while watching a two-year-old having a temper tantrum. Often the spark that set the conflagration off is lost to view or memory, but the toddler who is unable to make his opinion and feelings known through other and more socially acceptable ways can bring a family, a coach-load of people, a carriage in a train or a restaurant to a stunned silence. Then the feelings of anger spread and everyone around begins to hate the child and his mother and father, for not controlling the ridiculous outburst, and to resent the loss of time for their own affairs because of the disgusting and unasked-for intervention. Anger is without any doubt a very great force which seems to be built-in to each person at an early stage; but perhaps for many people the power and useful potential of this power remain either hidden or worse as a self-inhibiting or even self-destructive force. Our present society provides few outlets for this sort of strong feeling and the acceptable ways of controlling it could be paralysing for the development of the person.

It may be worth considering here that if the same toddler had fallen and cut himself he would most probably have received sympathy and attention and the onlookers would have been only too glad to help. I wonder if the hurt feelings or the hurt body actually give the small child greater distress; but the hurt body gets him comfort while the hurt feelings only get him a reprimand. Perhaps some of us learn early in our lives that cuts, bruises and other physical illnesses are tickets to receive some sort of comfort.

As the child grows he learns various ways of disguising his anger; and some of the disguises are very restrictive ones. If behaviour is all-important, real, and in particular, angry feelings may have to be hidden always or in some way covered up or changed into something else. What we say may always have to be different from what we really mean or feel. In the end we may no longer recognize our own anger. Ingrowing anger is a powerful force for harm to the owner and to all his relationships; and it is such a waste of talent that might have great potential for creation. Anger is a great power but it needs to be harnessed properly and not denied. To be of use it needs to be recognized, welcomed and then put to useful purposes.

Unhelpful ways of using anger

The toddler does not see himself as a monster although everybody else within earshot may well think of him as such. To the small child his parents, aunts, uncles or innocent bystanders are the monsters who are making his life infinitely unbearable. Fine, we may say that poor little child must grow up, learn better behaviour and get the world into better perspective. But is that what happens? Sadly, many people although looking adult and quite possibly appearing powerful and even pillars of the establishment still need to create their monsters. What about the intelligent but chronically depressed wife, who is chained to her house and her overbearing and demanding husband? She is as she is because of him or so she and everybody who knows her says. She is the victim. But is she? She chose to marry him so possibly she needs her husband as her own pet monster? Without him she might need to look at her own anger and inadequacies.

We all have our own monster-making machinery. And of course we are the victims of these terrible monsters. I enjoy Maurice Sendak's book *Where the Wild Things Are* and the opera which Oliver Knussen has created from it. These are the fantasies of the small child; but in real life they can continue their existence and cause wreckage for those who cannot recognize their private monsters as out-of-date and irrelevant to their current relationships. It is sad to see people going through the world re-creating their own early unhappy relationships with their fathers and mothers and blinkered to any way of creating a more loving present time. If you try to help you are all too likely to get caught up in their private monster-making machinery, and before you know where you are you have become one more monster. And you thought you were going to be a rescuer!

It can be very difficult to recognize that the anger and rage are in us and we must own them so that in the end we can tame them and use them productively. I believe that disowned or misplaced anger can sometimes have a lot to do with the onset and relapses in MS. The disease tends to occur in people who find it difficult to use their own strongest feelings in a creative way. It sometimes seems to me that MS is a disease much associated with anger and also the inability to handle anger constructively. When I reread the book about MS which I wrote ten years ago I recognize my own anger that MS was not diagnosed earlier and that it was misdiagnosed as a psychiatric illness. Surprisingly that no longer seems of such great importance to me.

Anger that can be owned and seen within us is a very useful emotion and can be harnessed to healing. It is only the unrecognized and hidden anger that is harmful. I sometimes fantasize that the geographical distribution of MS might be associated with the distribution of strong inhibitions on the showing of feelings including anger. Once again we need to think about the differences between correlations and associations and causes. I am not saying that anger causes MS but that a lot of inhibitions in showing strong feelings including anger may be associated with the development of MS and prevent its normal healing.

Ingrowing anger can be a most destructive emotion. It is recognized as playing a part in depression and depressive illnesses. But could feelings actually produce physical harm in the body? It has been noted that in the healthy breasts of many women whose bodies have been examined after death there can be small areas of 'cancer' but the areas have never developed into clinical cancer. Research has also been done on the relationship of breast cancer to certain sorts of stress. The same sort of thing could happen with MS-type lesions in the CNS. This is only speculation. It has been said that Nuclear Magnetic Resonance Imaging in the diagnosis of MS is too sensitive because it can sometimes pick up some hundreds of MS-like lesions. But what may happen, under certain conditions, perhaps even of acute tension, is that a lesion appears but mostly causes no clinical damage and is never recognized as disease. However, for some people more lesions appear and cause clinically recognizable MS. It may be more important to find out why these lesions develop and are important or why the lesions in other people do not develop and remain quiescent. It has been said that healing cannot occur in the CNS, but I have doubts about that. It may be necessary to know what prevents healing in the person who gets clinically recognizable MS.

Auto-immunity and anger

We have thought about auto-immunity and the body's recognition of its own tissues. An invader gets killed off but the body does not usually damage its own tissues. But under some conditions the body can and does do damage to itself. MS may be one of the illnesses in which the body fails to recognize itself and damages and destroys its own nervous tissue. I have wondered if this sort of destruction could be triggered by changes that take place in the body due to the physiological stresses that occur under tension. Ingrowing anger could perhaps be one of the major stresses. The twentieth century is a stressful time and perhaps we are beginning to see a new range of stress-related illnesses. Such illnesses may include new and more severe types of allergic illness.

Competitiveness that prevents healing

In present-day Western civilization we have to tolerate a high level of competitiveness. As babies we are quieter than or heavier than or sleep better than and so on. We then get better at work or slower at music or faster at running. In everything we are compared with someone else. So what happens if someone just cannot keep going in this artificial sort of race? Perhaps they have a mental breakdown: and that is not too socially acceptable. Or they might have a heart attack or develop another disease such as hypertension. The pressures of competition could favour keeping a disease, such as migraine or asthma, which may be a sort of personal and acceptable escape route when pressures become intolerable. Living in this sort of competitive environment could also prevent healing because healing needs time and peace and the release from pressure.

What are the optimum conditions for healing?

Having looked at some of the things that I believe can prevent a person's return to health, which is normal, we now need to think about the ways that can help that return. I must repeat that I do not know all the answers and am sure that I never shall. I can only try and write about the ways in which healing can occur in the light of my own experiences of the past two years. I do not pretend that I now have a new cure for MS. And I must stress yet again that I am not saying that MS is all in the mind, the result of malingering and not really a physical illness. I am beginning to think that there is no real division between diseases of the body, mind and spirit and it is only the present custom of doctors and scientists that keeps this artificial division; perhaps the time is coming when the essential one-ness of each person can be accepted.

At the time of writing the movement for holistic medicine is taking root. If doctors could understand and work with Christian humility and priests could take human anger on board and understand the power and potential of the subconscious mind there would be a real movement towards better understanding of health and disease. The concept of whole person disease must be understood from within the patient rather than decided from without. If it is decided by some powerful person that what I need is music therapy I do not believe that it will have the same long-term benefit on me and my disease as if I had discovered from within that I needed an outlet in music. Of course, it has traditionally been the role of the professional worker to see what others need, but I should prefer help in understanding what I need and then help in finding it. Doctors, nurses and other helpers and healers including priests can only be catalysts in the healing processes. I am sure now that a human being cannot be divided into body, mind and spirit but is an interlinked whole; any sickness is a varying amount of sickness of these three indissoluble parts. Perhaps when we can all understand this and the different role that any one of a number of helpers can give, we shall be nearer bringing peace and reconciliation to the warring components in each person who has dis-ease.

So what are the optimum conditions for healing?

A real desire for healing

Obviously the person with an illness will not say that he prefers to keep the illness rather than get better. That would look like some very strange sort of perversion. But he still may not want to change the things in his life that would enable healing to start. An obvious example is the man with severe bronchitis who will not give up smoking or understand what cigarettes are doing to his lungs and try to find a substitute comfort. He is happy to co-operate with the doctors and take his antibiotics and use oxygen but he refuses to take the most important, and for him painful, step and give up smoking.

Doctors tend to encourage this passive approach and collude with the patient who is happy to accept treatment in a passive manner and wait to be made better. It would be different if doctors and patients alike could begin to see that healing might be the norm and that everybody needs to think seriously about the optimum conditions in which normal healing can occur. At this point doctor and patient would become co-workers towards such healing and their roles would be changed to ones of total equality with the deciding vote on action in the patient's hand.

Before there can be an honest and wholehearted desire for healing the patient must be prepared to relinquish every possible gain from his illness. That means understanding the value of the extra attention, caring or sympathy that he gets because he is ill and then being prepared to give them all up. This sort of clear-sighted understanding of the self is difficult and it is always more comfortable to draw a few veils over some of our depths.

Dwelling on our present state of illness and unhappiness can prevent us from seeing the need to go forward. I have found it helpful to think in practical terms of life as a pilgrimage, of being held back or holding ourselves back by dwelling on the unhappiness or evil of the past, of the total awfulness of our parents, of the doctors who have wronged us and done us physical and mental harm. Actually our parents also had awful parents – and so have our children but the camouflage and fashions change. We just have to pick up our share of the burdens, forgive or try to forgive those we see as having wronged us and then stagger on. We are all on the same pilgrimage and we are not going to arrive yet. A pilgrimage is not a matter of scoring goals in a competitive way. It is more relevant to keep getting one foot in front of the other, physically and metaphorically. It is not a race to a triumphant arrival at the top of the stairs. If we are forever returning in thought to the past and lamenting the things that might have been we can remain oblivious to the things that could be.

The need to recognize the sickness within as well as outside

I am not using the word 'within' to mean the MS lesions which are hidden in the CNS, but in the sense of illness existing at different levels of one's being. I believe in many people with MS there is a warring component between the body, the mind and the emotions. There is often a part that is self-driving, ambitious, responsible, commanding and independent; but there is also the side that desperately needs to be cared for, nurtured and protected. The first or 'adult' self can so easily be led into a sort of warfare with the 'child' or dependent self. In so many MS patients the 'adult' part can become the carer and very much a needed person such as a doctor, nurse or teacher. As long as this part is in control the mind and body can work together in reasonable harmony and the flaws in the wholeness of the person do not become apparent. But when tension increases or control is threatened the flaws can become more apparent and I believe that the threat to the wholeness of the person may be the concealed anger. It is too dangerous to allow this anger out and therefore it is turned inwards.

The idea of the destructive power of ingrowing rage is not new to the psychiatrist, who may see it as a cause of depression. It is also familiar to the psychosexual counsellor who meets it as impotence in the male and loss of libido in the female. Often the cause of these problems is unrecognized, unexpressed and sometimes unexpressable rage with the sexual partner. We all know the phrase 'impotent rage'. During the past two years I have learned a great deal about the rage within myself which has contributed to my illness. As I have understood and recognized a little more of the rage, healing has occurred and is occurring. During the early months of my relapse I began to be aware of the physical feelings of rage particularly in my legs. It was worst in the general areas of the muscles that had been most affected. While I was trapped with my rage the weakness of my legs remained. And I was also aware of directing a lot of rage at my legs because they had let me down.

When I decided that I really did want to become as healthy as possible there were some difficult choices to be made. The biggest thing was practising clinical medicine. I had never done much full-time medical work but had come to enjoy it during the five years prior to my relapse. The thought of giving it up meant the relinquishment of something I had come to value, also of financial security and the sense of value that comes from knowing that you are giving help. The pain of losing these things was great but when I sorted out my priorities I knew that they must go before other things could be allowed to happen. For me it is always difficult to give up any present security because I find it difficult to trust in what may be going to happen unless I have firm control over it.

Giving up medicine was a part of my delivery from all the pressures that I had put on myself. It was also for me the beginning of delivery from the tyrant child within me, from many old fears, and from needs for pretence and possessions. It was also for me the beginning of daring to allow things to happen rather than plotting and planning to make them happen. This was, for me, a totally new attitude. To dare to wait and allow is very different from the will-power and manipulation involved in contriving to make something happen.

For me some of the blessings of giving up were very unexpected. It gave me time to share John's last year of life and perhaps most importantly his death. As a doctor I had seen many dead bodies but had never before shared anybody's death; and I found it strangely beautiful as well as sad. I realized that death was just one more marker on the way and not an end.

The importance of touch

I have thought a great deal about touch during the past two years and of its great importance in the process of healing. The medical 'licence to touch' has always been important in the doctor/patient relationship. But it goes far beyond this. I love the story in the gospels of the woman with an issue of blood. This is the version from the Jerusalem Bible. 'Now there was a woman suffering from a haemorrhage for twelve years, whom no one had been able to cure. She came up behind Jesus and touched the fringe of his cloak; and the haemorrhage stopped at that instant. Jesus said, "Who touched me?" When they all denied that they had, Peter and his companions said, "Master, it is the crowds round you, pushing." But Jesus said, "Somebody touched me. I felt that power had gone out from me." Seeing herself discovered, the woman came forward trembling, and falling at his feet explained in front of all the people why she had touched him and how she had been cured at that very moment. "My daughter," he said, "your faith has restored you to health; go in peace."' I think the woman must have had a heavy and continuous loss of blood from her uterus which can be caused by, as well as causing, great personal distress. It is fascinating to watch her comfort and healing from touch and Jesus' awareness of his 'power' that had gone to the woman in the touch.

At present there is much publicity about child sexual abuse. It will be a sad outcome from all the publicity if parents are inhibited in touching their own small children of both sexes. Women may touch and kiss both men and women in public, but in the UK it is not widely acceptable for men to touch and embrace each other. I sometimes wonder if men are not being needlessly deprived by this social taboo on touch of a gentle power that might reduce their aggression. Sadly the only embracing that does occur between men publicly at present is associated with scoring goals!

Two years ago a friend who was doing a course in therapeutic massage wanted a guinea-pig, saw that I was looking poorly and was confined more or less to the house because of my weak legs and asked if she could massage me. My own angry feelings about myself and my intense dislike of my body made it almost impossible for me to let her near enough for massage. However, she quietly persisted and eventually I managed to allow her to massage me although it made me feel frighteningly vulnerable. Her patience, acceptance and her remarkable hands began to lessen my loathing for my body. The massage also relieved much of the muscle spasm and tension in my body. Being massaged by somebody known and trusted is a good start to the building or rebuilding of a personal world of trust. Possibly other people with MS would find this sort of whole body massage healing.

I shall add here another piece of my jigsaw puzzle although I am not sure where it will fit. During the third week of the development of the human embryo there is a differentiation into three layers which are endoderm, ectoderm and mesoderm. The skin and nervous system develop from the same layer, the ectoderm. During the third week of intra-uterine life the ectoderm along the back of the embryo thickens and then extends into the interior of the embryo like a fold. This invagination becomes separated from the outer part of the ectoderm and a tube develops within the invaginated portion of the ectoderm. From this tube the nervous system develops. I am intrigued by the development of the skin and nervous system from the ectoderm and also by the close connections I have experienced between touching of the skin and healing of the nervous system.

Another way of using touch for healing is described by Father Robert Llewelyn in his book *A Doorway to Silence. The Contemplative Use of the Rosary*. Father Robert is an Anglican priest and now priest to the Julian shrine in Norwich. He can be best described as a holy and spiritual man and his spirituality somehow cannot be described as belonging to one part of the Christian church or perhaps not even to one sort of religion. I will write more about his suggested use of touch in the context of inner stillness.

I can so easily ignore the joys of ordinary touch in everyday life and this perpetual loss may be for me another way of preventing my own healing. I mean the feel of clothes that are made of cotton, wool or silk that I prefer next to my skin. I like the feel of cool cotton or linen sheets when I get into bed, and lying in warm water in the bath. I enjoy a regular treat of swimming in an indoor and adequately heated swimming-pool and then ten minutes in the solarium. I have found out that this is not carcinogenic and I only do it once a fortnight; but for me this is healing. I enjoy the feel of rain and wind and sunshine on my skin. I could go on but the reader will be able to think of other and more relevant pleasures to be found by touching. I believe that the conscious selection and positive enjoyment of these sensations is both healing in the general sense but more particularly is important for the healing of the nervous system in MS.

The acceptance and healing use of anger

I have only had glimpses of the right ways in which anger can be harnessed and used. Too often I still misuse it and do harm to myself and also to close friends and my family. Nobody can doubt the extra-ordinary intensity and power of anger, as we have already seen in the tantrums of a small child.

Anger and its creative and healing powers can only become good influences when you are able to accept them as your own. I must learn to understand and accept my own anger before I can use it creatively in living and loving. It is going to take more than my lifetime to acquire such wisdom. It can never be my mother or my husband or my boss who made me become what I am; because I am now an adult and as powerful – and as angry – as they are. If I wish to remain in the position of a child and a maker of monsters, I can, but then I must be prepared to accept all the misery, confusion, insecurity and unhappiness of the dependent child. This is comparable to the traditional patient role but I can change this if I really want to. There are disadvantages as well as advantages in choosing to become an adult and leave the child behind but at least if I am able to do that I shall have more choice.

I am writing this book on a word processor and when I look at some of the 'exit' options on offer which include 'cancel' and 'abandon' I think of anger. Perhaps cancel and abandon would be good ways to let outdated and irrelevant anger go away from us.

So often I have found in the past two years that the answer to a problem is either within me or else very close at hand. It is not something 'out there' that is being denied me by some powerful person or circumstances beyond my control.

This is a place to include a few quotations from the writings of Julian of Norwich which I have found of particular help in the past two years. They are nearly all from *Enfolded in Love* published by Darton, Longman & Todd. The one most relevant to the ownership of anger is:

> I saw full surely that wherever our Lord appears, peace reigns, and anger has no place. For I saw no whit of anger in God – in short or in long term.

> The best prayer is to rest in the goodness of God, knowing that goodness can reach right down to our lowest depths of need.

> And when we have fallen, through frailty or blindness, then our courteous Lord touches us, stirs and calls us. And then he wills that we should see our wretchedness and humbly acknowledge it. But it is not his will that we should stay like this, nor does he will that we should busy ourselves too much with self-accusation; nor is it his will that we should despise ourselves. But he wills that we should turn quickly to him.

> Though we are in such pain, trouble and distress, that it seems to us that we are unable to think of anything except how we are and what we feel, yet as soon as we may, we are to pass lightly over it and count it as nothing. And why? Because God wills that we should understand that if we know him and love him and reverently fear

him, we shall have rest and be at peace. And we shall rejoice in all he does. He did not say, 'You shall not be tempest-tossed, you shall not be work weary, you shall not be discomforted.' But he said, 'You shall not be overcome.' God wants us to heed these words so that we shall always be strong in trust, both in sorrow and in joy.

God is the still point at the centre.

Because of our good Lord's tender love to all those who shall be saved, he quickly comforts them saying, 'The cause of all this pain is sin. But all shall be well, and all shall be well, and all manner of thing shall be well.'

A prayer I have found helpful but not attributed to Julian of Norwich is:

So easily do we pray for the wrong things:
For strength that we may achieve, and God gives us weakness that we may be humble;
For health that we may do great things, and God gives us infirmity that we may do better things;
For riches that we may be happy, and God gives us poverty that we may be wise;
For power that we may have the praise of men, and God gives us weakness that we may feel the need of him;
For all things that we may have life, and God gives us life that we may enjoy all things.
And so having received nothing that we have asked for but all things that we have genuinely hoped for, our prayer has been answered, and we have been blessed.

The practice of stillness

The pressures of modern life and the seductions of the consumer society are very great. There are forces at work on all of us wanting us to conform to an image depending on our sex, age, etc. There are enormous pressures particularly on the young to conform in matters of hairstyle, entertainment, music, clothes, and so on. But there are pressures on most of us: the pressures on the middle-aged to have the right sort of holidays, cars and houses, pressures on doctors to make acceptable diagnoses, pressures to 'succeed' in competitive environments. All these pressures are very much on the outside and urge us to conform from the outside in. Everything, including illnesses and the treatment for them has to be packaged, classified and labelled. But people are essentially not packageable. They are unique and everything I am trying to say in this book is about a respect for the uniqueness of each one of us, an individual approach to sickness and the need for healing to start at the centre – not at the outside. For someone with MS, it is important when he thinks about the healing process starting at the centre, to look at his attitude to himself. If healing has to start at the centre, diet and routines of rest and exercise will assume a greater importance because they are part of a new spirit of caring for the self.

Greed may be another impediment to healing. To be healthy we need to have good relationships with God (or our spiritual equivalent) our neighbours, ourselves and creation. Scoring points on the size of our houses, the distance from home and the cost of our holidays, and so on, does not help us towards inner peace and stillness, but we have to accept the sort of society in which we live. We all need regular doses of the grace of God or some kind of spiritual strength because nothing good is possible in our strength alone. It is up to us to find ways of finding and accepting this medicine. We can find it in our own way and in our own time. I am not suggesting that practising contemplation is the new cure for MS; what I am saying is that it has been profoundly helpful for me and in many unexpected and surprising ways. Perhaps a miracle is just something beyond our present expectations and we need to remain full of expectant prayer.

I shall include here some quotations from Father Robert Llewelyn's book *A Doorway to Silence. The Contemplative Use of the Rosary*. You do not have to be a Roman Catholic to use a rosary. It can be a useful way of stilling the restless mind, body and spirit for any who choose to use it. If you find these ideas interesting I suggest you buy his book and read more about it.

The rosary and the sense of touch

A valuable focus of attention as you say the rosary is one part or another of your own body. You say the words of the Hail Mary which help to relax the mind but your attention is focused gently on a part of your body.

Obviously it makes special sense to direct the attention to the fingers holding the beads. As you hold each bead and say the Hail Mary your awareness goes into the sense of touch experienced by your fingers. Nothing exists for you for the moment but this feeling of the fingers on the bead. All heaven and earth is gathered into it. As your attention strays you bring it gently back.

The rosary is healing

But your awareness need not go into your fingers. You can go round the whole body, making each part an object of attention or awareness, saying the rosary prayers at the same time. Thus, be aware of the heart centre. As you say the prayer, look gently towards it in the mind. Let your mind descend into the heart. You are directing the healing energy of love to that part of your body.

Then go round your body, mentally taking one or two beads for each part. Take whatever part occurs to you: the shoulders, the arms, the hands; the brow, the face, the jaw. Through your awareness of these parts direct the healing energy of love to each in turn. So far as time allows do not leave anything out.

In this way you bring healing to every part of yourself, that body-soul-spirit complex which makes up each one of us.

Perhaps one half of the hospital beds in the country would be emptied if everyone were to spend fifteen minutes on this each day (or on any other exercise in this book). Personally I believe it would be more than half.

And what a boon to the Health Service, and to every other service too. No government, of whatever party, can create a welfare state if we, the people, are failing to draw upon the spiritual resources available to us.

I feel sure that the Secretary of State for Health and Social Services might find the free issue of rosaries and Father Robert Llewelyn's book as a new way of cutting costs in the financially overstretched Health Service rather surprising!

A reconciliation of our warring bodies, minds and spirits is essential before there can be any real stillness within us. We need to accept the child, and possibly a very angry and disruptive child within us. We may not like that bit of us but if we have to keep this part of us hidden from our view at all times we can stop some sort of healing energy being allowed to flow through us. The need to hide this angry child and keep it out of sight at all times can also make us very frightened of losing control in any way.

Another book I have found helpful is *Heaven in Ordinary. Contemplative Prayer in Ordinary Life* by Angela Ashwin (Mayhew McCrimmon). Here is an exercise from this delightful book:

An Exercise with a Marble
Try this! If you have lots to do in a short time, try an exercise with a marble. Before you rush to do the next job, STOP, just for a moment. (This seems daft because it cuts down the time you have even more. But try it.) Your mind is probably buzzing with all that needs doing, like a marble rolling round a large wooden bowl. Stop and picture that marble going round and round, gradually coming to the centre of the bowl, and stopping there, remaining quite still. Let your own mind, like the marble, slow down and stop at this central point, which is where you are here and now. You are now ready to do the job with the whole of yourself and not just a harassed part of your mind (while the rest of your thoughts were racing around incontrollably). Your mind is quiet and you can concentrate fully on the task in hand. Now get to work! If you wish, you can decide which job you will do after this one. But plan no farther ahead than that. Don't let the marble start rolling around again.

Here is another exercise which I have found extraordinarily helpful for encouraging me to allow things to happen rather than making things happen, which is my more habitual way of behaving. It comes from *Becoming a Writer* by Dorothea Brande (Macmillan Papermac). She writes:

This is a very simple but rather spectacular experiment which you can make that will teach you more about your own processes of putting an idea into operation than pages of exhortation and explanation. It is this: Draw a circle on a sheet of paper, using the bottom of a tumbler or something of that circumference as the guide; then make a cross through it. Tie a heavy key on a string about four inches long. Hold the end of the string with the ring hanging like the weight of a pendulum over the intersection of the cross, about an inch above the paper. Now THINK around the circle, following the circumference with your eyes and ignoring the ring and cord entirely.

After a few moments the little pendulum will begin to swing around in the direction you have chosen, at first making a very small circle, but steadily widening as it goes on. Then reverse the direction in thought only and follow the circle with your eyes in the other direction . . . Now think up and down the perpendicular line; when that succeeds, shift to the horizontal. In each case the ring will stop for a moment and then begin to move in the direction of your thinking.

If you have not tried this experiment before you may feel that there is something uncanny about the result. There isn't. It is simply the neatest and easiest way of showing how important imagination can be in the sphere of action. Minute involuntary muscles take up the task for you. The will, you see, was hardly involved in the matter at all. And this, some French psychologists say, is the way to observe, in miniature, a 'faith cure' in operation. At the least, it should demonstrate that it is not necessary to brace every nerve and muscle to bring about a change in your daily life.

This was written by an American woman writer and teacher of creative writing and first published in 1934, republished in 1982. The book is definitely not connected with MS, but I have found that exercise so useful and I believe that if MS patients could learn something about allowing things to happen and relying to a much greater extent on their subconscious energy, MS fatigue might be more manageable. You have to learn to trust and allow something to happen and not in true MS fashion contrive and manipulate to MAKE it happen. It is so much easier for me to write about this than to learn to live it!

Who are the healers?

I have always had some unpleasant gut reaction about the phrase 'I am a Healer' but I had never really thought about the problem clearly. I am sure that there are people with special psychic gifts of healing, but I am equally certain that anyone can be a healer and at most times is one. I have big doubts about the use of capital letters as used in Healer or Ministry of Healing. Yes, I am sure, as stated in the gospels,

Christians were sent out to heal the sick but I think that it was a completely normal part of Christian life and life could be lived in the same way now. But perhaps before that there are many other things which need to happen such as selling all our goods and giving to the poor and holding all things in common. I feel certain that there must be complete humility about any acts of healing and the 'healer' is only a sort of catalyst or heavenly midwife delivering the sick person from sickness, and not as having achieved anything in his own right and power; and there must never be an unseemly display of the scalps of the healed!

However, there are holy men and women in our midst who are able to show the love of God with total humility. One of my helpers has been a wise old priest with whom I have been totally honest and able to talk freely about the unspeakable. He can in his radiance and utter humility help me to understand a little about God's love and about human love. The acceptance of the unacceptable, the loving of the loathsome, of trust and of reconciliation. He was able to throw the first rope across my personal chasm between the horrors of the needy and the security and safe position of the needed. Out of his love and humility, which always make him stress that his powers are not of himself, I began to understand the power of love which can accept all things not necessarily with human approval but with understanding. For me that meant a greater understanding of hope for the hopeless, faith for the faithless, trust for the untrusting and love for the loveless, unloved and apparently unlovable. For other MS patients and their families and friends who have another type of faith my particular path will be of no significance. For those who do not have any sort of faith there may be other, different and effective understanding but perhaps a more difficult puzzle for those whose understanding includes only the body and the mind.

Hope for the future

My orthodox medical training and work will always remain a part of me and I still look critically at 'alternative' or 'complementary' medicine. But I know that my own healing has not been through orthodox channels only. I shall remain in a state of unknowing about healing – and about Christianity. However, I can say with conviction that I was sick and I am now being healed. I do not know how it has happened but I know that it is happening. I hope that for the last years of my life my body will be an adequate tool because this is a time when I want to be able to concentrate less on physical things.

Appendix   Sources of Help

Health problems

The Social Worker

The social worker is based in the hospital or the community and is the first person to contact. She will be able to inform the MS patient and her family about other sources of help available locally, both in the statutory and voluntary sectors. She will be able to make contact with other workers if required to and advise on available financial assistance.

The Nurse

A nurse in either the hospital or community service will be able to help in many ways including ordinary nursing care, emotional support and education.

The Health Visitor

The health visitor may be contacted through the GP and can help with many general problems of the family and patient. She does not do ordinary practical nursing.

The Occupational Therapist

The OT, based in the hospital or community, can work with the physiotherapist in helping a person with MS manage everyday needs in the home. She is also able to arrange necessary alterations to a home, supply mobility aids and give help about employment.

The Physiotherapist

She will be hospital- or community-based and more is written about her work on pp.66–70.

The Speech Therapist

The speech therapist can help with problems of speech, language and swallowing.

Help with employment

Manpower Services Commission can help with finding work for disabled people and can be contacted through the local Job Centre.

The Disablement Resettlement Officer can also be contacted through the local Job Centre and will give information about all the available help for disabled people.

Home Opportunities for Professional Employment, 19 Langland Gardens, London NW3 6QE.

Association of Disabled Professionals, c/o The Stables, 73 Pound Road, Banstead, Surrey SM7 2HU.

Legal problems

Citizens Advice Bureaux. Local addresses will be found in the telephone directory.

Network for the Handicapped, 16 Princeton Street, London WC1R 4BB.

Welfare benefits

Full information about the benefits currently available can be obtained from the local office of the Department of Health and Social Security at the address in the local telephone directory.

Mobility

Information about help available may be obtained from the local or central MS Society, the local DHSS office or the Disability Alliance.

Housing

Information about Housing Benefit can be obtained from the local DHSS office.

Information about grants to adapt and improve houses can be obtained from the local authority or the occupational therapist.

Further reading

McAlpine's Multiple Sclerosis by Matthews, Acheson, Batchelor and Weller, Churchill Livingstone. (A medical textbook obtainable through a reference library)

Multiple Sclerosis: Immunological, Diagnostic and Therapeutic Aspects, edited by F. Clifford Rose, John Libbey. (A medical textbook obtainable through a reference library)

Multiple Sclerosis: The Facts, by W. B. Matthews, Oxford University Press

Multiple Sclerosis by Bernie O'Brien, Office of Health Economics

Multiple Sclerosis: Psychological and Social Aspects, edited by A. Simons, Heinemann Medical Books

Multiple Sclerosis: A Personal Exploration by Alexander Burnfield, Souvenir Press

Multiple Sclerosis. A Self-help Guide to Its Management by Judy Graham, Thorsons

Multiple Sclerosis: A Guide for Patients and their Families by L. Scheinberg, Raven Press, New York, USA

Learning to Live with Multiple Sclerosis by R. Povey, R. Dowie, G. Prett, Sheldon Press

Multiple Sclerosis. Control of the Disease by W. Ritchie Russell, Pergamon Press

Yoga for the Disabled by Howard Kent, Thorsons

Yoga for Handicapped People by B. Brosnan, Souvenir Press

Physical Fitness developed by the Royal Canadian Air Force, Penguin

The Complete Scarsdale Medical Diet by H. Tarnower and S. S. Baker, Bantam Books

The Dieter's Guide to Success by A. Byton and H. Jordan, Fontana

A Doorway to Silence by Robert Llewelyn, Darton, Longman & Todd

Enfolded in Love. Daily Readings with Julian of Norwich, Darton, Longman & Todd

Directory of Aids for Disabled and Elderly People edited by Ann Darnbrough and Derek Kinrade, Woodhead-Faulkner

Useful Addresses

The Multiple Sclerosis Society of Great Britain and Northern Ireland, 25 Effie Road, Fulham, London SW6 1EE. Tel: 01 736 6267

MS Society in Scotland, 27 Castle Street, Edinburgh, Midlothian EH2 3DN. Tel: 031 225 3600

MS Society in N. Ireland, 34 Annadale Avenue, Belfast BT7 3JJ. Tel: 0232 644914.

ARMS (Action for Research into Multiple Sclerosis), 11 Dartmouth Street, London SW1H 9BL. Tel: 01-222 3224

ARMS Research Unit, Central Middlesex Hospital, Acton Lane, Park Royal, London NW10. Tel: 01-961 4911

International Federation of Multiple Sclerosis Societies, 3/9 Heddon Street, Suite 22, London W1R 7LE.

RADAR (Royal Association for Disability and Rehabilitation), 25 Mortimer Street, London W1N 8AB.

For psychosexual problems:
Institute of Psychosexual Medicine, 11 Chandos Street, London W1M 9DE.

SPOD (Sexual and Personal Relations of the Disabled), 286 Camden Road, London N7 OBJ.

The Disabled Living Foundation, 380/384 Harrow Road, London W9 2HU.

The Disability Alliance, 25 Denmark Street, London WC2H 8NJ.

Yoga for Health Foundation, Ickwell Bury, Northill, Biggleswade, Bedfordshire.

Addresses for MS in the USA

National Multiple Sclerosis Society, 205 East 42nd Street, New York NY 10017

National Committee for Research on Neurological and Communicative Disorders, 1120 20th Street, N.W. Suite 201, Washington, DC 20036

Disability Rights Center, 1346 Connecticut Ave. N.W. Suite 1124, Washington, DC 20036

American Coalition of Citizens with Disabilities, 1200 15th Street, N.W. Suite 201 Washington, DC 2005

Information Center for Individuals with Disabilities, 20 Providence Street, Room 329, Boston, MA 02196

Independent Citizens Research Foundation for the Study of Degenerative Diseases, P.O. Box 97, Ardsley, NY 10502

Addresses for MS in Australia

National Multiple Sclerosis Society of Australia, 616 Riversdale Road, Camberwell, Vic. 3124

Multiple Sclerosis Society of Queensland, P.O. Box 370, Woolloongabba, Qld. 4102

Multiple Sclerosis Society of New South Wales, P.O. Box 364, Artarmon, N.S.W. 2064

Multiple Sclerosis Society of Victoria, 616 Riversdale Road, Camberwell, Vic. 3124

Multiple Sclerosis Society of South Australia & N.T. Inc., P.O. Box 198, Greenacres, S.A. 5086

Multiple Sclerosis Society of W.A. (inc.), P.O. Box 1168, Victoria Park East, W.A. 6101

Multiple Sclerosis Society of Tasmania, P.O. Box 213, North Hobart, Tas. 7002

National Multiple Sclerosis Society of New Zealand Room 501, Bonaventure House, Wellington N3

Acknowledgements

Thanks are due for permission to quote from the following works:

Robert Llewelyn, *A Doorway to Silence*, Darton, Longman & Todd Ltd, 1986
Enfolded in Love: Daily Readings with Julian of Norwich, Darton, Longman & Todd Ltd, 1980
Dorothea Brande, *Becoming a Writer*, Papermac, 1983
Audrey Eyton and Henry Jordan, *The Dieter's Guide to Success*, Fontana, 1981

Index

ACTH, 10, 20, 30, 45
AIDS, 30
anger, 13, 17, 22, 36, 120–4, 129–31
ARMS, 47, 55, 67, 68
auto-immune disease, 30, 123, 124
azathioprine, 46

benign MS, 11, 14, 15, 27
bereavement, 76, 77
bladder problems, 35, 99–101
bowel problems, 101

cerebro-spinal fluid, 29, 33, 37, 38, 39, 46
Charcot, 27
clumsiness, 9, 12, 35
competitiveness, 124
constipation, 101
contemplation, 133, 134
contraception, 91
corticosteroids, 45
CT scanning, 9, 39, 41, 45
curing of disease, 114

death, 128
dementia, 105
demyelination, 33, 40, 41, 42, 100, 101
depression, 36, 99, 104, 123, 127
diagnosis, 9, 10, 37–42

diet, 9, 32
double vision, 6, 34

EEG, 39
ejaculatory problems, 90
embryology, 129, 130
essential fatty acids, 32, 55
essential fatty acid diet, 60, 61
euphoria, 36
evening primrose oil, 32, 55
evoked potentials, 39
exercise, 68–70

falling over, 101–3
fats, saturated and unsaturated, 32, 54
fatigue, 7, 11, 15, 36, 71–5, 82–4, 94, 104
financial worries, 17, 87, 95
food allergies, 63

general practitioner, 107
genetic factors, 31, 93
geographical distribution, 27, 28
giddiness, 35
gluten-free diet, 62, 63
greed, 133

healers, 136, 137
healing of disease, 114, 116–38
herpes simplex, 30
HLA system, 31

hobbies, 96
hyperbaric oxygen, 46–8

immunity, 31
immuno-gamma globulin, 40
immunosuppression, 46
impotence, 90, 91, 127
incontinence, 100
investigations, 37–42

Julian of Norwich, 131, 132
journalism, 96, 97

linoleic acid, 32
low-fat diet, 53–60
lumbar puncture, 9, 39, 40

malaria, 9
massage, 129
measles antibody, 29
metrizamide myelography, 39, 40
monster-making, 121, 122, 131
multifactorial causes, 29
MS Society, 15, 55
muscle cramp, spasms and
    twitching, 20, 36, 98, 129
myelin sheath, 33

nerve, 33
neurologist, 13, 14, 20, 27, 108
neurosis, 11, 77
NMRI, 39, 41, 42
nocturnal erections, 91

occupation and MS, 94–7
optic nerve and neuritis, 34, 41,
    45, 99
orgasm, 91

pain, 99

physiotherapy, 66–70
pilgrimage, 126
Poser Committee Diagnostic
    Guides, 37
pregnancy, 6, 92, 93
psychiatric illness, 7, 11, 19

Randomized Controlled Trial,
    43, 44
relapse, 18
rest, 72, 73
Rosary, use of, 130, 133, 134

Scarsdale diet, 52
secondary gain from illness, 118,
    119, 126
sensation, 35
signs, 33
speech difficulty, 36
stillness, the practice of, 132–6
sugar, 50, 51, 61
Swank, Dr R., 32, 54
symptoms, 33

touch, 128–30
trigeminal neuralgia, 99

urgency, 100

vegan diet, 63
virus, 29, 33
vision, 6
vitamin and mineral supplements,
    55, 63, 64, 65

weakness, 6, 7, 19, 34
weight loss, 9, 51–4

yoga, 70
yoghurt, 60